KETO BREAD

COOKBOOK

COMPLETE STEP-BY-STEP GUIDE TO COOKING HEALTHY DISHES BREAD WITH THE KETOGENIC DIET

Susan Blunder

TABLE OF CONTENTS

INTRODUCTION

Congratulations on purchasing *Keto Bread Cookbook,* and thank you for doing so. The following chapters will discuss the benefits of enjoying ketogenic bread, what to eat, and what to avoid on the keto plan, what tools you will need for baking, and so much more. You will have tons of options to choose from, whether it is a loaf of bread or a delicious cookie.

Each delicious bread recipe has full instructions, the time needed to prepare, nutritional information, and how many servings you will be preparing.

A Bit Of History

Before we begin, let's decide why keto's history proves it is not a fad diet plan. During the 1920s and 1930s, the ketogenic diet was used medically for its role in epilepsy therapy treatments as an alternative method - versus the uncharacteristic fasting methods used. It was victorious in the treatment plan's early phases.

However, during the 1940s, the keto dieting process was abandoned because of new and improved therapies discovered for those who suffered from seizures. Approximately 20-30% of the epileptic cases during that time had failed to control seizures. With that failure, the ketogenic diet was reintroduced as a management technique.

As time passed, the Charlie Foundation was founded by the family of Charlie Abraham in 1994 after Charlie's recovery from seizures and other health issues he suffered daily. As a youngster, Charlie was placed on the diet and continued to use it for five years. As of 2016, he was still functioning successfully without the seizure episodes and was furthering his education as a college student.

In 2006, The Charlie Foundation appointed a panel of dietitians and neurologists to agree in an official statement. It was written as an approval of the dieting techniques and stated which cases its use would be considered. It is noted that the plan is especially recommended for children. This was just the beginning.

Bread Baking Basics

Let's look at the basics of how you will prepare your delicious bread using the keto plan.

Mixing the Recipe: You will be taking raw ingredients from a recipe. In the case of bread, it will consist mainly of water, flour, yeast, and salt. Next, mix them to form the dough.

Proofing The Bread: Proofing is the baking phase where the yeast eats the flour's sugars. The result is that it burps out alcohol and built-up gases, which causes the bread to rise and gives it a natural and sweet flavor.

Baking Delicious & Healthy Bread At Home: You are 'proofing' and nurturing the dough so you can prepare a healthy meal for your family. Your primary goal is to achieve a tasty loaf of bread that looks and tastes like it came from a professional bakery.

Baking the Bread: Baking is considered the stage where you apply the hot oven to your masterpiece. You will be creating a tasty treat.

Storing & Eating: The final phase is the easiest; just serve and enjoy the bread.

Get The Right Water And Flour Ratio

If you are following a recipe, you will have the correct ratios for preparing your bread. However, if you decide seven or eight cups isn't precise enough, the process works like this. Most sandwich bread is 2:1 flour to water. Therefore, if your dough seems to be sticky, don't be tempted to add more flour to the mixture. The result could be a loaf that will not rise.

If you don't want to take a chance of adding too much flour when preparing the work surface, you can use a light mist of cooking spray or a small amount of olive oil. You can also use some water to prevent sticky issues. Using a bench scraper, you can easily remove the dough off of the preparation surface.

Temperature is Important

It is essential to pay close attention to the temperatures when combining the ingredients into your bread. All recipe components should be around the 68-70° Fahrenheit temperature range. This method helps keep the dough 'stretchy' to rise to its expected potential.

Generally speaking, proteins (such as eggs) take longer to incorporate if they are too cold. If the product is too warm, it can also lose its elasticity. The fat should be moldable and soft such as the texture of Play-Doh - malleable and not melty. You shouldn't be able to run your fingers through it.

These are a few pointers, so you better organize your work area and make your first successful keto bread for your friends or family. I hope you will enjoy each segment of the book and will better understand how to make delicious and healthier bread choices while on the ketogenic diet plan.

Now, sit back and relax; enjoy the journey to ketosis using these delicious bread options!

CHAPTER 1

BUN SPECIALTIES

Almond Buns For Sandwiches

Servings Provided: 6

Prep & Cook Time: 25-28 minutes

Macro Counts - Per Serving:

- Calories: 199

- Net Carbohydrates: 4.2 g

- Fat Content: 19 g

- Protein: 5.2 g

Essential Ingredients:

- Almond flour (1 cup)

- Large eggs (3)

- Butter (2 oz.)

- Salt (1 pinch)

- Baking powder (1 tsp.)

Preparation Technique:

1. Heat the oven to reach 380° F/194° C.

2. Add the eggs to a mixing container and whisk.

3. Melt the butter in a pan or the microwave and add to the eggs and whisk again.

4. Combine all of the fixings, gently folding by hand.

5. Arrange in the baking pan.

6. Bake for about 15 minutes.

BREAKFAST BUNS

Servings Provided: 4

Prep & Cook Time: 45 minutes

Macro Counts - Per Serving:

- Calories: 309

- Net Carbohydrates: 4 g

- Fat Content: 26 g

- Protein: 9.4 g

Essential Ingredients:

- Almond flour (.75 cup)

- Baking powder (1 tsp.)

- Psyllium husk powder (2 tbsp.)

- Salt (.5 tsp.)

- Shelled sunflower seeds (1 tbsp.)

- Whole flaxseeds (1 tbsp.)

- Eggs (2)

- Olive oil (2 tbsp.)

- Sour cream (.5 cup)

Preparation Technique:

1. Set the oven temperature to reach 400° F/204° C.

2. Prepare a cake pan using a layer of parchment baking paper.

3. Mix the dry fixings (psyllium, flour, baking powder, salt, and seeds).

4. Combine the eggs with the sour cream and oil. Fold into the dry fixings. Let it stand for five minutes.

5. Slice the dough into four portions and shape into a ball.

6. Arrange the balls in the prepared pan.

7. Bake them until browned to your liking (20 to -25 min.).

GARLIC & BASIL BUNS

Servings Provided: 8

Prep & Cook Time: 35-40 minutes

Macro Counts - Per Serving:

- Calories: 186

- Net Carbohydrates: 1.4 g

- Fat Content: 15 g

- Protein: 9.6 g

Essential Ingredients:

- Salt (1 pinch)

- Water (.75 cup)

- Butter (6 tbsp.)

- Almond flour (.75 cup)

- Chopped fresh basil (1 cup)

- Garlic (6 cloves)

- Eggs (4)

- Parmesan (5.5 oz)

Preparation Technique:

1. Heat the oven to reach 400° F/204° C.

2. Chop the basil, grate the parmesan, and crush the garlic cloves.

3. Cover a baking tray using a layer of parchment baking paper.

4. Boil the water and add the salt and butter.

5. Transfer the pan to a cool burner and whisk in the flour. Combine well, and break in the eggs.

6. Fold in the garlic, basil, and lastly - the parmesan.

7. Once it's creamy, add the dough onto the prepared pan - one spoonful at a time while shaping into buns.

8. Bake for 20 minutes and enjoy. Cool before storing.

GARLIC HOT DOG BUNS

Servings Provided: 20

Prep & Cook Time: 1 hour 10 minutes

Macro Counts - Per Serving:

- Calories: 92

- Net Carbohydrates: 1 g

- Fat Content: 9 g

- Protein: 2 g

Essential Ingredients:

- Ground psyllium husk powder (5 tbsp.)

- Baking powder (2 tsp.)

- Sea salt (1 tsp.)

- Almond flour (1.25 cups)

- White/cider vinegar (2 tsp.)

- Boiling water (1 cup)

- Egg whites (3) The Garlic Butter:

- Unchilled butter (4 oz.)

- Garlic (1 clove)

- Fresh parsley - finely chopped (2 tbsp.)

- Salt (.5 tsp.)

Preparation Technique:

1. Set the oven temperature to 400° F/204° C.

2. Cover a baking tray with a layer of parchment paper.

3. Boil the water and add the salt and butter.

4. Transfer the pan to the countertop and add the flour.

5. Combine thoroughly, and break in the eggs. Be sure to combine the eggs thoroughly before adding the next one.

   (It's a critical step.)

6. Mince and fold in the garlic, basil, and lastly - the parmesan.

7. Once it's creamy, add the dough on the prepared pan - one spoonful at a time while shaping into buns.

8. Bake for 20 minutes and serve. Cool before storing.

HEALTHY SPRING ONION BUNS

Servings Provided: 6

Prep & Cook Time: 40 minutes

Macro Counts - Per Serving:

- Calories: 81

- Net Carbohydrates: 1.1 g

- Fat Content: 6.7 g

- Protein: 4.2 g

Essential Ingredients:

- Separated eggs (3)

- Stevia (1 tsp.)

- Cream cheese (3.5 oz.)

- Baking powder (.5 tsp.)

- Salt (1 pinch) *The Filling:*

- Chopped hard-boiled egg (1)

- Diced spring onions (2 sprigs)

Preparation Technique:

1. Set the oven temperature setting to reach 300° F/149° C.

2. Spritz the muffin cups with a bit of oil.

3. Whisk the egg yolks with the stevia, cream cheese, baking powder, and salt. Whisk the egg whites in another cup.

4. Combine the fixings with a spatula, and add the dough to the muffin cups.

5. Combine the filling components and add them to the cups.

6. Scoop more dough into the cup. It's important to fill the cups only half full to allow room for the rest of the fillings. Bake for 30 minutes.

7. Cool slightly to serve.

KETO POPPY SEED BUNS

Servings Provided: 12

Prep & Cook Time: 35 minutes

Macro Counts - Per Serving:

- Calories: 162

- Net Carbohydrates: 6 g

- Fat Content: 11.5 g

- Protein: 11 g

Essential Ingredients:

- Salt (.5 tsp.)

- Psyllium husk powder (.33 cup)

- Coconut flour (.5 cup)

- Almond flour (2 cups)

- Cream of tartar (2 tsp.)

- Garlic powder (2 tsp.)

- Baking soda (1 tsp.)

- Eggs (6 whites & 2 whole)

- Boiling water (2 cups)

- Poppy seeds (2 tbsp.)

Preparation Technique:

1. Set the oven temperature setting to reach 350° F/177° C.

2. Combine all of the dry fixings.

3. In another mixing container, whisk and add all of the eggs. Pour in the boiling water and continue stirring. Combine everything and stir until mixed well.

4. Spoon into the pan. Bake for 20 to 25 minutes.

KETO SESAME BUNS

Servings Provided: 12

Prep & Cook Time: 1 hour 5 minutes

Macro Counts - Per Serving:

- Calories: 133

- Net Carbohydrates: 4 g

- Fat Content: 6.5 g

- Protein: 7 g

Essential Ingredients:

- Egg whites (8)

- Baking powder (1 tbsp.)

- Psyllium powder (.5 cup)

- Coconut flour (1 cup)

- Hot water (1 cup)

- Sesame seeds (.5 cup + .5 cup to cover the buns)

- Pumpkin seeds (.5 cup)

- Sea salt (1 tbsp.)

- Boiling water (1 cup)

Preparation Technique:

1. Set the oven in advance to reach 350° F/177° C.

2. Blend the egg whites in a blender until foamy.

3. Combine the dry fixings in a food processor until crumbly.

4. Pour in the water and stir to create a smoother dough.

5. Make 12 buns. Empty the additional ½ cup sesame seeds in a dish and cover the top side of the bun.

6. Arrange the buns on a parchment paper-covered baking sheet to bake for 50 minutes.

PROTEIN SOYA BUNS

Servings Provided: 8

Prep & Cook Time: 45 minutes

Macro Counts - Per Serving:

- Calories: 29

- Net Carbohydrates: 0.1 g

- Fat Content: 0.3 g

- Protein: 6 g

Essential Ingredients:

- Oil for the holders

- Eggs (2)

- Water (.5 cup)

- Soya protein powder (1.5 or 2 oz.)

- Vanilla extract (.125 tsp.)

- Cinnamon (.125 tsp.)

- Stevia (1 dash)

Preparation Technique:

1. Heat the oven to reach 425° F/218° C.

2. Prepare the baking cups with a spritz of oil.

3. Whisk the eggs and add the rest of the fixings.

4. Portion the prepared batter into the cups.

5. Bake for 20 minutes. Lower the setting to 340° F/171° C.

6. Bake for another 10 to 15 minutes to serve.

ULTIMATE KETO BUNS

Servings Provided: 6

Prep & Cook Time: 32 minutes

Macro Counts - Per Serving:

- Calories: 230

- Net Carbohydrates: 1.8 g

- Fat Content: 20.8 g

- Protein: 8.5 g

Essential Ingredients:

- Melted lard/unsalted butter/beef tallow (4 tbsp.)

- Eggs (4)

- Himalayan salt (.5 tsp.)

- Blanched almond flour (1 cup)

- Black sesame seeds (1 tbsp.)

- Rosemary (1 tbsp.)

- Onion flakes (1 tsp.)

- White sesame seeds (1 tbsp.) *Also Needed*:

- Stick blender with beaker

- Silicone jumbo muffin molds (6)

Preparation Technique:

1. Heat the oven in advance to 430° F/221° C.

2. Add the eggs and melted lard/butter inside the stick blender beaker.

3. Add the rest of the fixings over the liquid.

4. Pulse with the stick blender inside the beaker five to ten times until all of the batter is thoroughly mixed. Pour the mixture into the molds.

5. Sprinkle a few sesame seeds over the buns as desired.

6. Set the timer and bake for 26 minutes. Transfer the pan from the oven and let the buns thoroughly cool before slicing.

7. Notes: If you want a thicker bun, pour the batter into four molds instead of six.

8. Once cooled, just add them to a zipper-type bag and put them in the fridge for another time. The buns are even tastier the following day.

9. Freeze them - making sure to slice the bun first.

VEGAN BURGER BUNS

Servings Provided: 6

Prep & Cook Time: 50 minutes

Macro Counts - Per Serving:

- Calories: 182

- Net Carbohydrates: 6.4 g

- Fat Content: 10.3 g

- Protein: 6 g

Essential Ingredients:

- Coconut flour fresh - lump-free (1 cup)

- Ground psyllium husk (.25 cup)

- Almond meal (.5 cup)

- Olive or vegetable oil of choice (2 tbsp.)

- Baking soda (2 tsp.)

- Lemon juice/Apple cider vinegar (2 tsp.)

- Sea salt (.25 tsp.)

- Water (1.75 cups)

Preparation Technique:

1. Set the oven temperature setting to 400° F/204° C.

2. Prepare a baking tray with a layer of parchment baking paper. Spritz with cooking oil spray.

3. In a mixing bowl, whisk all of the dry ingredients.

4. Add in the rest of the fixings, and stir vigorously with a spatula at first, for about ½ minute. Knead the dough for an extra one minute.

5. Set aside for ten minutes in the mixing container. This step is crucial for the fiber to absorb the extra moisture from the psyllium husk to create a soft elastic dough.

6. Knead the dough for ½ minute and divide it into six balls. Arrange them on the prepared tray, leaving at least one thumb between each of the buns.

7. Press each ball to flatten slightly and shape into a bun. Brush a tiny amount of water on the top of each of the buns and garnish using sesame seeds.

8. Bake the buns for 20-25 minutes using the oven's center level until the top is crispy and browned to your liking.

9. Cool for 20 minutes. Slice in half using a bread knife.

CHAPTER 2

LOAF BREAD SPECIALTIES

ALMOND CHIA LOW-CARB BREAD

Servings Provided: 12

Prep & Cook Time: 1 hour 8 minutes

Macro Counts - Per Serving:

- Calories: 107

- Net Carbohydrates: 2.4 g

- Fat Content: 6.3 g

- Protein: g

Essential Ingredients:

- Greek yogurt (1 cup)

- Eggs (3)

- Almond flour (1 cup)

- Baking powder (.5 tbsp.)

- Coconut flour (2 tbsp.)

- Psyllium husks (3 tbsp.) *or* husk powder (1.5 tbsp.)

- Chia seeds (3 tbsp.)

- Salt (.5 tsp.)

- *Optional:* Sunflower seeds (2 tbsp.)

- *Also Needed*: Small loaf pan

Preparation Technique:

1. Prepare the loaf pan using a layer of parchment baking paper.

2. Blend the yogurt and eggs using an electric mixer.

3. Mix in coconut flour, almond flour/ground almonds, baking powder, and salt. Mix until thoroughly combined.

4. Fold in the psyllium husks, chia seeds, and sunflower seeds.

5. Choose a warm space to store the bowl of dough so it can rise for about 15 minutes. Sprinkle using the sunflower seeds.

6. Heat the oven to reach 340° F/171° C. Set a timer and bake for 45 minutes. Serve when it is browned to your preference.

7. *Note*: For the almond flour, you can substitute almond meal or ground almonds.

BROWN KETO BREAD

Servings Provided: 16

Prep & Cook Time: 1 hour 20 minutes

Macro Counts - Per Serving:

- Calories: 137

- Net Carbohydrates: 1.9 g

- Fat Content: 8.8 g

- Protein: 12 g

Essential Ingredients:

- Sugar or inulin (2 tbsp.)

- Salt (1 pinch)

- Baking powder (1 tsp.)

- Almond flour (2.5 cups)

- Whey protein isolate (2 cups)

- Xanthan gum (1 tbsp.)

- Instant yeast (1 tsp.)

- Warm water (1.25 cups)

- *Also Needed*: 9 by 5-inch loaf pan

Preparation Technique:

1. Warm the oven before baking time to reach 375° F/191° C. Lightly spritz the loaf pan with cooking oil or use a sheet of parchment baking paper.

2. Whisk the dry fixings, including the instant yeast.

3. Slowly pour in warm water and whisk until it's a thick batter-type consistency. Scoop the batter into the pan.

4. Put a kitchen tea towel over the pan and place it in a warm place to rise until the dough doubles in size (45 minutes).

5. Sprinkle water over the dough tops and bake the bread for 20-25 minutes. Serve hot.

CAULIFLOWER BREAD

Servings Provided: 10

Prep & Cook Time: 1 hour 10 minutes

Macro Counts - Per Serving:

- Calories: 204

- Net Carbohydrates: 4 g

- Fat Content: 17 g

- Protein: 7 g

Essential Ingredients:

- Riced cauliflower (3 cups)

- Eggs (6 large - separated)

- Olive oil (6 tbsp.)

- Baking powder (1 tbsp.)

- Super-fine almond flour (1.25 cups)

- Salt (1 tsp.)

- *Also Needed*: 8 x 8-inch loaf pan

Preparation Technique:

1. Set the oven temperature at 350° F/177° C.

2. Prepare the pan using parchment paper.

3. Finely chop the cauliflower and microwave the cauliflower for three to four minutes or until tender. Let it cool and place a small amount in a tea towel and wring it dry. Repeat with remaining cauliflower, working in small batches.

4. Add the egg whites into a mixing container. Blend until stiff peaks form using the high-speed setting of an electric mixer. Set aside.

5. Combine the egg yolks, oil, baking powder, almond flour, and salt. Mix to create a smooth paste. Stir in the cauliflower until evenly mixed.

6. Fold the egg whites into the paste. When the egg whites are completely folded in, add in another batch, and repeat until all of the egg whites are incorporated.

7. *Note*: Be careful not to beat the egg whites because that will cause them to lose the air-whipped into them, and the bread will not properly rise.

8. Dump the mixture into the prepared pan.

9. Bake for about 45 to 50 minutes. Cool before slicing.

COCONUT BREAD

Servings Provided: 8

Prep & Cook Time: 50-55 minutes

Macro Counts - Per Serving:

- Calories: 161

- Net Carbohydrates: 3 g

- Fat Content: 13 g

- Protein: 5 g

Essential Ingredients:

- Eggs (6)

- Coconut oil (.33 cup)

- Unsweetened almond milk (.33 cup)

- Salt (.25 tsp.)

- Xanthan gum (1 tsp.)

- Coconut flour (.5 cup)

- Baking powder (1 tbsp.)

Preparation Technique:

1. Set the oven to reach 350° F/177° C.

2. Spray a pan using a cooking oil spray.

3. Whisk the coconut oil, milk, and eggs.

4. Fold in salt, coconut flour, and baking powder. Stir until it's thickened, and dump into the pan.

5. Set the timer and bake for 35-45 minutes. Wait just a few minutes before serving.

COCONUT ALMOND FLOUR BREAD

Servings Provided: 8

Prep & Cook Time: 50-55 minutes

Macro Counts - Per Serving:

- Calories: 161

- Net Carbohydrates: 3 g

- Fat Content: 13 g

- Protein: 5 g

Essential Ingredients:

- Eggs (6)

- Coconut oil (.33 cup)

- Unsweetened almond milk (.33 cup)

- Salt (.25 tsp.)

- Xanthan gum (1 tsp.)

- Coconut flour (.5 cup)

- Baking powder (1 tbsp.)

Preparation Technique:

1. Warm up the oven to reach 350° F/177° C.

2. Whisk the coconut oil with the milk and eggs.

3. Sift and mix in the baking powder, coconut flour, and salt.

4. Stir until it has thickened.

5. In a greased bread pan, spread the mixture evenly.

6. Bake for 35 to 40 minutes.

7. Allow the bread to cool slightly before serving.

COCONUT-FLAXSEED BREAD

Servings Provided: 8

Prep & Cook Time: 45-50 minutes

Macro Counts - Per Serving:

- Calories: 183

- Net Carbohydrates: 3.2 g

- Fat Content: 14 g

- Protein: 1 g

Essential Ingredients:

- Coconut flour (.75 cup)
- Ground flaxseed or flax meal (.5 cup)

- Large eggs (3)
- Large egg whites (3)
- Olive oil (5 tbsp.)
- Baking powder (2 tsp.)
- Water (10 tbsp.)
- Sea salt (1 pinch)

Preparation Technique:

1. Warm the oven to reach 350° F/177° C.

2. Spritz a baking pan with cooking oil spray.

3. Combine the egg whites and eggs with a processor or electric mixer until foamy. Add the remainder of the fixings until the dough is smooth.

4. Wait for about four to five minutes, so the flax and coconut flours can absorb the moisture.

5. Arrange the dough into the baking tray and bake until it's browned.

6. Notes: Times vary; 25-30 minutes for the loaf or approximately 35 minutes or for muffins.

FLAX & ALMOND BREAD

Servings Provided: 8 - varies

Prep & Cook Time: 20 minutes

Macro Counts - Per Serving:

- Net Carbohydrates: 6 g

- Protein: 14 g

- Fat Content: 42 g

Ingredients:

- Almond meal/almond flour (35 g)

- Flaxseed meal/whole ground flaxseed (40 g)

- Baking powder - ex. - Calumet/Magic brand - Kraft (4 g)

- Salt (1.5 g)

- Vinegar, white distilled (any brand (2 g)

- Liquid Stevia - ex. - NOW Stevia (4 drops)

- Raw mixed egg (85 g)

- Melted - coconut oil (31 g) or butter (37 g)

- Also Needed: 8 x 8-inch pan

Preparation Technique:

1. Heat the oven to 350° F/177° C.

2. Weigh all ingredients and combine the dry ones first. Then mix in the wet ones.

3. Lightly grease the baking pan and add the bread.

4. Bake for eight to ten minutes. Slice with a knife and lift it from the pan with a spatula.

FLAXSEED BREAD

Servings Provided: 12

Prep & Cook Time: 35-38 minutes

Macro Counts - Per Serving:

- Calories: 185

- Net Carbohydrates: 0.7 g

- Fat Content: 7.5 g

- Protein: 6 g

Essential Ingredients:

- Baking powder (1 tbsp.)

- Flaxseed meal (2 cups)

- Salt (1 tsp.)

- Olive oil (.33 cup)

- Water (.5 cup)

- Whisked eggs (5)

- Maple syrup (1-2 tbsp.)

- 10 by 15-inch baking pan with sides

Preparation Technique:

1. Heat the oven in advance to reach 350° F/177° C.

2. Lightly oil a sheet of baking paper or use a mat.

3. Whisk all of the dry fixings. Mix with the rest of the wet components. After the bread dough is formed, let it rest for two to three minutes to thicken.

4. Pour into the oiled pan, pulling it away from the center for more even baking results. Stretch it into a rectangular shape, leaving about two inches from the end of the pan.

5. Bake until it has visibly browned (24-28 min.). It's entirely done when it springs back to the touch.

GARLIC BREAD

Servings Provided: 20

Prep & Cook Time: 1 hour 10 minutes

Macro Counts - Per Serving:

- Calories: 92

- Net Carbohydrates: 1 g

- Fat Content: 9 g

- Protein: 2 g

Essential Ingredients:

- Almond flour (1.25 cups)

- Baking powder (2 tsp.)

- Ground psyllium husk powder (5 tbsp.)

- Sea salt (1 tsp.)

- White wine or cider vinegar (2 tsp.)

- Boiling water (1 cup)

- Egg whites (3) The Garlic Butter:

- Unchilled butter (4 oz.)

- Garlic clove (1 minced)

- Fresh parsley - finely chopped (2 tbsp.)

- Salt (.5 tsp.)

Preparation Technique:

1. Set the oven to reach 350° F/177° C. Combine the dry fixings in a mixing container.

2. Start a pot of water. Once boiling, pour in the egg whites and vinegar. Whisk using a hand mixer for about ½ minute.

3. Shape and roll into hot dog-size buns, leaving plenty of space to allow for expansion.

4. Bake using the lower rack for 40-50 minutes. When ready, remove to cool.

5. Mince the garlic and prepare the garlic butter to chill.

6. Slice the cooled buns using a serrated knife and spread garlic butter on each half. Reheat the oven to 425° F/218° C.

7. Bake until lightly browned (10-15 minutes).

MACADAMIA BREAD

Servings Provided: 16

Prep & Cook Time: 50 minutes

Macro Counts - Per Serving:

- Calories: 227

- Net Carbohydrates: 5 g

- Fat Content: 22 g

- Protein: 5 g

Essential Ingredients:

- Macadamia nuts (2 cups)

- Eggs (4)

- Almond flour (.25 cup)

- Sea salt (1 tsp.)

- Ground flaxseed (2 tbsp.)

- Softened ghee (.25 cup)

- Softened coconut butter (.5 cup)

- Baking powder (.5 tsp.)

- Apple cider vinegar (2 tbsp.)

- Also Needed:

- Food processor & an 's' blade

- 8 by 4-inch loaf pan

Preparation Technique:

1. Set the oven temperature to 350° F/177° C.

2. Lightly grease the pan with ghee.

3. Process the nuts using the food processor until they are a fine flour.

4. Add the eggs - 1 at a time - with the motor running until the mixture is creamy.

5. Fold in the flaxseed, almond flour, coconut butter, ghee, vinegar, sea salt, and baking powder. Continue processing until well combined.

6. Scoop in the oiled bread pan.

7. Bake for 35-40 minutes.

8. Cool the bread before slicing to serve or store.

SAVORY STUFFED BREAD

Servings Provided: 10

Prep & Cook Time: 1 hour

Macro Counts - Per Serving:

- Calories: 202

- Net Carbohydrates: 2 g

- Fat Content: 20 g

- Protein: 6 g

Essential Ingredients:

- Baking powder (1.5 tsp.)

- Parsley seasoning (2 tbsp.)

- Sage (1 tsp.)

- Rosemary (1 tsp.)

- Medium eggs (8)

- Cream cheese (1 cup)

- Butter (.5 cup)

- Almond flour (2.5 cups)

- Coconut flour (.25 cup)

Preparation Technique:

1. Set the oven temperature at 350° F/177° C.

2. Grease a loaf pan.

3. Cream the butter, cream cheese, sage, parsley, and rosemary.

4. Whisk and break in the egg to create the batter. Stir until it's smooth.

5. Combine the almond and coconut flour with the baking powder.

6. Mix all of the fixings until well incorporated. Scoop into the loaf pan.

7. Bake for 50 minutes and serve.

SESAME SEED BREAD

Servings Provided: 6

Prep & Cook Time: 1 hour 30 minutes

Macro Counts - Per Serving:

- Calories: 100

- Net Carbohydrates: 1 g

- Fat Content: 13 g

- Protein: 7 g

Essential Ingredients:

- Baking powder (2 tsp.)

- Almond flour (1.25 cups)

- Sesame seeds (2 tbsp.)

- Psyllium husk powder (5 tbsp.)

- Sea salt (.25 tsp.)

- Apple cider vinegar (2 tsp.)

- Boiling water (1 cup)

- Egg whites (3)

- Also Useful: Hand mixer

Preparation Technique:

1. Warm the oven temperature to reach 350° F/177° C.

2. Spritz a baking tin with cooking oil spray. Put the water in a saucepan to boil.

3. Combine the almond flour, baking powder, sea salt, sesame seeds, and psyllium powder.

4. Stir in hot water, vinegar, and egg whites. Use a hand mixer (less than 1 min.) to combine. Place the bread on the prepared pan.

5. Bake for one hour on the lowest rack. Serve and enjoy any time.

SOURDOUGH BREAD

Servings Provided: 8 slices

Prep & Cook Time: 1 hour 10 minutes

Macro Counts - Per Serving:

- Calories: 317

- Net Carbohydrates: 4 g

- Fat Content: 22 g

- Protein: 11 g

Essential Ingredients:

Dry Components:

- Almond flour (1.5 cups)

- Coconut flour (.5 cup)

- Flaxseed meal (.5 cup)

- Baking soda (1 tsp.)

- Salt (1 tsp.)

- Psyllium powder (.33 cup)

- Citric acid (.5 tsp.) *Wet Components*:

- Egg whites (6)

- Eggs (2 whole)

- Heavy whipping cream (.5 cup)

- Boiling water (BOILING a must) (.75 cup)

- Apple cider vinegar (.25 cup)

Preparation Technique:

1. Heat the oven at 350° F/177° C.

2. Measure and add all of the dry ingredients into a mixing container. Pour in *boiling* water and combine until uniform. (Boiling water activates Psyllium husk powder.)

3. Use another mixing container, whisk and add all of the eggs, whipping cream, and cider vinegar.

4. Add the egg mixture to the dry ingredient and water mixture. Combine until uniform. You might need to use your hands.

5. Scoop the dough onto a baking sheet covered with a sheet of parchment baking paper. Shape the dough into a round ball.

6. Score the top of the dough with an "x" shape for a nice top.

7. Bake until golden brown (45-50 min.). If you tap it on it lightly and get a hollow sound, your bread is done.

8. Place the bread onto a wire rack to cool.

9. Slice to serve, but don't slice until it's had a while to cool.

10. Toast if desired.

WALNUT BREAD

Servings Provided: 10

Prep & Cook Time: 1 hour 13 minutes

Macro Counts - Per Serving:

- Calories: 269

- Net Carbohydrates: 11 g

- Fat Content: 22 g

- Protein: 8 g

Essential Ingredients:

- Coconut oil (for the pan)

- Olive oil (.25 cup)

- Bananas (3 medium)

- Eggs (3 large)

- Walnuts (.5 cup)

- Baking soda (1 tsp.)

- Almond flour (2 cups)

Preparation Technique:

1. Set the oven temperature setting to 350° F/177° C.

2. Lightly grease a loaf pan with the coconut oil.

3. Slice the bananas into circles. Toss them into a mixing container with the rest of the fixings. Use the blender (high setting) to prepare the batter.

4. Empty the prepared batter into the greased loaf pan.

5. Set a timer to bake the bread for about 50 minutes to one hour.

6. Cool slightly. Serve warm if desired.

CHAPTER 3

BISCUIT & ROLL SPECIALTIES

BISCUITS

ALMOND DROP BISCUITS WITH CHEESE

Servings Provided: 6

Prep & Cook Time: 15-20 minutes

Macro Counts - Per Serving:

- Calories: 144

- Net Carbohydrates: 2 g

- Fat Content: 13 g

- Protein: 5 g

Essential Ingredients:

- Baking powder (1 tbsp.)

- Salt (1 pinch)

- Baking soda (.5 tsp.)

- Almond flour (1.5 cups)

- Eggs (2 whole)

- Sour cream (.5 cup)

- Melted grass-fed butter (4 tbsp.)

- Shredded cheddar cheese (.5 cup)

- Swerve confectioners (1 tsp.)

- Baking spray (as needed)

Preparation Technique:

1. Set the oven temperature to reach 450° F/232° C.

2. Prepare a muffin pan with liners or spritz the pan with a little cooking oil spray.

3. Use a hand mixer or whisk to mix the baking powder, salt, almond flour, and baking soda.

4. Whisk the eggs with the swerve, sour cream, and melted butter.

5. Combine all of the fixings. Scoop the batter directly into the baking pan.

6. Bake for 9-12 minutes. Cool slightly to serve.

BACON CHEDDAR DROP BISCUITS

Servings Provided: 10

Prep & Cook Time: 30 minutes

Macro Counts - Per Serving:

- Calories: 154

- Net Carbohydrates: 2 g

- Fat Content: 14 g

- Protein: 6 g

Essential Ingredients:

- Bacon (4 slices)

- Baking powder (1 tbsp.)

- Almond flour (1.5 cups)

- Dried parsley (1 tbsp.)

- Baking soda (.5 tsp.)

- Garlic salt (1 tsp.)

- Onion powder (1 tsp.)

- Eggs (2)

- Sour cream (.5 cup)

- Bacon grease melted (1 tbsp.)

- Shredded cheddar cheese (.33 cup)

- Shredded smoky bacon cheddar cheese (.33 cup)

- Melted grass-fed butter (3 tbsp.)

- Swerve confectioners/powdered erythritol (.5 tsp.)

Preparation Technique:

1. Warm the oven in advance at 425° F/218° C.

2. Prepare a baking pan using a sheet of parchment paper.

3. Fry and crumble the bacon.

4. Whisk the baking powder, almond flour, onion powder, garlic salt, and baking soda into a mixing container.

5. Combine the eggs, melted butter, bacon, parsley, bacon grease, and sour cream.

6. Mix in the cheese and combine everything. Scoop the biscuit mixture onto the prepared pan.

7. Bake for 11-15 minutes and serve.

FLUFFY ALMOND FLOUR BISCUITS

Servings Provided: 7

Prep & Cook Time: 20 minutes

Macro Counts - Per Serving:

- Calories: 151

- Net Carbohydrates: 1.4 g

- Fat Content: 15 g

- Protein: 4 g

Essential Ingredients:

- Almond flour (1 cup)

- Melted butter/ghee (.125 cup)

- Egg (1)

- Salt (.5 tsp.)

- Pepper (.25 tsp.)

- Garlic powder (.25 tsp.)

- Baking soda (.5 tsp.)

- Apple cider vinegar (.5 tbsp.)

- *Optional*: Loosely packed basil (.5 cup) *or* Matcha (.5 tsp.) *or* your favorite herbs and spices

Preparation Technique:

1. Set the oven to reach 350° F/177° C. Prepare a baking tray using a parchment baking paper layer.

2. Whisk each of the fixings together in a large mixing dish (see the note below).

3. Scoop the dough and shape it into seven balls. Arrange onto the baking sheet, and flatten slightly.

4. Bake until golden and soft on the inside or for 15 minutes.

5. Transfer the biscuits to a cooling rack. Enjoy them warm.

6. *Note*: If using basil or Matcha, blend with almond flour in a blender until well mixed. Then, proceed to make the batter. Add in more almond meal (1-3 tbsp.) as needed until it forms a workable dough.

BREAKFAST LAVENDER BISCUITS

Servings Provided: 6

Prep & Cook Time: 30 minutes

Macro Counts - Per Serving:

- Calories: 270

- Net Carbohydrates: 4 g

- Fat Content: 25 g

- Protein: 10 g

Essential Ingredients:

- Coconut oil (.33 cup)

- Almond flour (1.5 cups)

- Egg whites (4)

- Kosher salt (1 pinch)

- Baking powder (1 tsp.)

- Culinary grade lavender buds (1 tbsp.)

- Liquid stevia (4 drops)

Preparation Technique:

1. Heat the oven to 350° F/177° C.

2. Spritz a baking sheet with a little coconut oil.

3. Combine the almond flour and coconut oil in a mixing container until it's pea-sized pieces. Set the bowl aside in the fridge.

4. Whisk the eggs until they start foaming. Toss in the salt, lavender, and baking powder. Stir well and mix in the eggs. Mix in with the almond mixture, stirring well.

5. Place the biscuits onto the baking sheet using an ice cream scoop or tablespoon. Pat them, so they aren't round, similar to a pancake.

6. Bake for 20 minutes and serve.

BUTTERY GARLIC & SHARP CHEDDAR BISCUITS

Servings Provided: 8

Prep & Cook Time: 35 minutes

Macro Counts - Per Serving:

- Calories: 144

- Net Carbohydrates: 0.5 g

- Fat Content: 12.8 g

- Protein: 6.7 g

Essential Ingredients:

- Garlic powder (.25 tsp.)

- Salt (.25 tsp.)

- Eggs (4)

- Butter (.25 cup)

- Baking powder (.25 tsp.)

- Sifted coconut flour (.33 cup)

- Shredded sharp cheddar cheese (1 cup)

Preparation Technique:

1. Set the oven temperature to 400° F/204° C.

2. Cover a baking tin using a sheet of aluminum foil and lightly grease with a spritz of oil.

3. Whisk the eggs with the garlic powder, butter, and salt. Whisk and fold in the baking powder and flour, whisking until the lumps are removed. Stir in the cheese.

4. Drop by the scoopful onto the baking pan.

5. Bake for about 15 minutes.

6. Leave the biscuits in the pan to cool for five to ten minutes. Transfer to a serving container.

CHEDDAR BAY BISCUITS

Servings Provided: 6

Prep & Cook Time: 15-20 minutes

Macro Counts - Per Serving:

- Calories: 216

- Net Carbohydrates: 2 g

- Fat Content: 19 g

- Protein: 9 g

Essential Ingredients:

- Finely ground/sifted almond flour (.75 cup)

- Dried parsley flakes (1 tbsp.)

- Baking powder (1.5 tsp.)

- Fine-grain salt (.5 tsp.)

- Garlic powder or granulated garlic (.5 tsp.)

- Sharp cheddar cheese (3 oz. - shredded)

- Large egg (1)

- Sour cream (.25 cup)

- Melted unsalted butter (2 tbsp.)

Preparation Technique:

1. Arrange the center-most oven rack in place. Heat the oven to reach 400° F/204° C.

2. Whisk the almond flour in with the baking powder, dried parsley, salt, and garlic powder in a large mixing bowl. Toss in the shredded cheese, mixing well.

3. Fold in the sour cream, egg, and melted butter.

4. Divide the batter mixture into six portions and place it on a lined half-sheet pan.

5. Bake until golden brown or for 10-13 minutes.

6. Allow cooling (2-3 min.) before serving. Serve warm.

SOUR CREAM BISCUITS

Servings Provided: 10

Prep & Cook Time: 25 minutes

Macro Counts - Per Serving:

- Calories: 189

- Net Carbohydrates: 3.2 g

- Fat Content: 16 g

- Protein: 6 g

Essential Ingredients:

- Hemp seed (2 tbsp.)

- Almond flour (1.5 cups)

- Baking powder (2 tsp.)

- Coconut flour (.33 cup)

- Salt (.5 tsp.)

- Swerve (1 tsp.)

- Baking soda (.5 tsp.)

- Sour cream (.5 cup)

- Egg (1)

- Melted butter (2 tbsp.)

- Cream (2 tbsp.)

- Water (2 tbsp./as needed)

Preparation Technique:

1.   Warm the oven to reach 450° F/232° C. At the same time, heat an iron skillet in the oven.

2.   Whisk the hemp seeds with the almond flour, baking soda, salt, coconut flour, baking powder, and sweetener.

3.   Whisk the egg with the cream, sour cream, melted butter, and water.

4.   Combine all of the fixings using gentle strokes. Set to the side for now.

5.   Measure and add the butter/bacon grease into the hot skillet.

6.   Arrange each of the biscuits in the skillet and transfer the skillet to the oven.

7.   Bake them for 11-15 minutes.

8.   Transfer to the countertop. Be sure to cool for about ten minutes before serving.

9.   Serve warm with a serving of butter or favorite low-carb toppings.

ROLLS

ALMOND & SOUR CREAM DINNER ROLLS

Servings Provided: 6

Prep & Cook Time: 35 minutes

Macro Counts - Per Serving:

- Calories: 277

- Net Carbohydrates: 3 g

- Fat Content: 26 g

- Protein: 9 g

Essential Ingredients:

- Almond flour (1.5 cups)

- Baking powder (2 tsp.)

- Salt (.5 tsp.)

- Sour cream (.33 cup)

- Melted butter (4 tbsp.)

- Eggs (2 large)

Preparation Technique:

1. Warm the oven to 390° F/199° C. Grease six wells of a square muffin tin.

2. Whisk the baking powder, almond flour, and salt. Add the sour cream, butter, and eggs and mix into a thick batter.

3. Spoon the batter evenly between the six holes.

4. Bake for 12 to 15 minutes or until the buns spring back when touched.

5. Wait for ten minutes and dump onto a rack to finish cooling.

CREAM CHEESE BREAD ROLLS

Servings Provided: 6

Prep & Cook Time: 1 hour 5 minutes

Macro Counts - Per Serving:

- Calories: 234

- Net Carbohydrates: 3 g

- Fat Content: 21 g

- Protein: 6 g

Essential Ingredients:

- Almond flour - blanched (1.25 cups)

- Psyllium husk powder (2-5 tbsp.)

- Celtic sea salt (1 tsp.)

- Baking powder (1 tsp.)

- Cream cheese (4 oz.)

- Butter (3 tbsp.)

- Boiling water (1 cup)

- Large egg (1)

Preparation Technique:

1. Set the oven temperature at 350° F/177° C.

2. Combine the dry fixings (psyllium, flour, baking powder, and salt). Set to the side for now.

3. In another glass dish, soften the cream cheese and butter in the microwave (or on the stovetop in a saucepan). Once it's glossy, remove from the burner/microwave and let it cool for about two minutes.

4. Add in and whisk the eggs until creamy. Stir in the rest of the ingredients to make the dough.

5. Use a measuring cup to scoop the dough onto a parchment-lined baking tray. Make six rolls using the dough.

6. Bake for 45-55 minutes and let it cool. Slice the cooled bread using a serrated knife.

7. Serve as it is or with a sandwich.

EGGLESS VEGAN BREAD ROLLS

Servings Provided: 6

Prep & Cook Time: 50 minutes

Macro Counts - Per Serving:

- Calories: 203

- Net Carbohydrates: 4.7 g

- Fat Content: 15 g

- Protein: 6 g

Essential Ingredients:

Dry Components:

- Almond flour (1.25 cups)

- Coconut flour (.25 cup)

- Ground psyllium husk (.25 cup + 3 tbsp.)

- Salt (.5 tsp.)

- Baking powder (2 tsp.) *Wet Fixings*:

- Olive oil (1 tbsp.)

- Apple cider vinegar (2 tsp.)

- Hot water - approx. 104° F/40° C (1 cup)

- *Optional Toppings*: Sesame seeds (2 tbsp.)

Preparation Technique:

1. Set the oven temperature in advance to 375° F/191° C.

2. Line a baking tray using a sheet of baking paper.

3. Whisk all the dry ingredients first.

4. Add the vinegar and olive oil. Stir in hot water. Combine for 1 minute to make the bread dough. Form a ball with your hand. (Don't add more than 1 tbsp. of husk.) Set aside for at least ten minutes to let the fiber absorb some of the liquid. The dough should be elastic, soft, and easy to divide into six small balls.

5. Roll each of the balls and place them onto the baking tray. They won't expand while baking. Brush the tops using a bit of tap water. Garnish using sesame seeds as desired.

6. Bake 40-45 minutes at the very bottom of the oven for ½ hour. Change the pan to the top level of the oven for 10-15 minutes.

7. For crusty bread, turn on the grill mode for an extra five minutes after the 45 minutes of baking.

8. Fully cool down a cooling rack before serving.

GARLIC & CHEDDAR FATHEAD DOUGH DINNER ROLLS

Servings Provided: 8

Prep & Cook Time: 35 minutes

Macro Counts - Per Serving:

- Calories: 230

- Net Carbohydrates: 3 g

- Fat Content: 16 g

- Protein: 12 g

Essential Ingredients:

- Cheddar cheese grated (8 oz.)

- Butter (2 tbsp.)

- Coconut flour (.5 cup)

- Baking powder (4 tsp.)

- Unflavored whey/egg white protein powder (.25 cup)

- Garlic powder (1 tsp.)

- Salt (.25 tsp.)

- Whole large eggs (2)

- Large egg white (1)

- *Also Needed*: 8-inch round baking pan *The Garlic Butter:*

- Melted butter (2 tbsp.)

- Garlic cloves (2 minced)

- Freshly chopped parsley (1 tbsp.)

- Coarse salt (.5 tsp.)

Preparation Technique:

1.   Set the oven in advance at 350° F/177° C.

2.   Line the baking pan with a sheet of baking paper.

3.   Using a microwave-safe bowl, combine the grated cheese with the butter. Melt it using high in 30-second increments until the cheese and butter can be stirred together easily.

4.   Mix in the protein powder, baking powder, coconut flour, garlic powder, and salt. Stir in all of the eggs and egg white.

5.   Use a rubber spatula for kneading it together in the bowl until uniform.

6.   Portion the dough into eight balls, and place in the baking pan.

7.   Whisk the fixings for the garlic butter. Brush about half of it over the rolls in the pan.

8.   Bake until firm when lightly touched and puffy (20-25 min.).

9.   Remove and wait for about 15 minutes before removing from the pan and breaking apart.

10. Brush with the remaining garlic butter. Serve warm.

HAWAIIAN ROLLS

Servings Provided: 12 rolls

Prep & Cook Time: 1 hour 40 minutes

Macro Counts - Per Serving:

- Calories: 197

- Net Carbohydrates: 2 g

- Fat Content: 17 g

- Protein: 9 g

Essential Ingredients:

- Almond flour (1 cup)

- Golden erythritol (.33 cup)

- Coconut flour (3 tbsp.)

- Baking powder (4 tbsp.)

- Xanthan Gum/flax powder substitute - if needed (1 tsp.)

- Mozzarella (2 cups - shredded)

- Cream cheese (8 oz.)

- Eggs (3 large)

- Pineapple flavoring (.5 tsp.)

- Suggested 11x7-inch baking dish

Preparation Technique:

1.   Add all of the dry ingredients into a large mixing container and stir until combined.

2.   Whisk and mix the eggs and pineapple flavoring to the dry fixings, but don't over mix.

3.   Warm the mozzarella and cream cheese in a large microwave-safe container using 30-second intervals mixing at each pause until thoroughly combined.

4.   Combine the cheese mixture to the dough and mix until combined. Use oiled hands if needed to "knead" the dough.

5.   Set the oven temperature to reach 350° F/177° C.

6.   Pour oil into the baking dish. Using your hands, roll the dough into 12 balls.

7.   Place the dough balls onto the baking tray - slightly separated.

8.   Place a layer of foil over the dish. Set a timer and bake for 40-45 minutes.

9.   Discard the foil, brush with melted butter, and bake it for another 15-20 minutes, until the rolls are browned and have a hollow sound when tapped.

10. Let cool for ten minutes and separate the rolls with a knife.

11. Store in a closed container for four to five days.

PARMESAN GARLIC KNOTS

Servings Provided: 8 @ 2 each portion

Prep & Cook Time: 35 minutes

Macro Counts - Per Serving:

- Calories: 220

- Net Carbohydrates: 2.7 g

- Fat Content: 19 g

- Protein: 7 g

Essential Ingredients:

- Almond flour (.5 cup)

- Garlic powder (.5 tsp.)

- Coconut flour (.25 cup)

- Baking powder (2 tsp.)

- Salt (.25 tsp.)

- Shredded part-skim mozzarella cheese (1.5 cups)

- Melted butter (5 tbsp.)

- Large egg (1) *The Butter:*

- Butter - melted (3 tbsp.)

- Parmesan cheese (2 tbsp.)

- Garlic (2 tsp.)

- Kosher salt (.75 tsp.)

- Dried parsley (.5 tsp.)

Preparation Technique:

1. Warm the oven to reach 350° F/177° C.

2. Prepare a baking tray using a silicone liner or baking paper. Mince the garlic and grate the parmesan, and set aside for now.

3. Whisk the almond flour with the garlic powder, baking powder, coconut flour, and salt.

4. Melt the cheese in a saucepan using the low-temperature setting until it can be easily stirred. Mix in the butter and egg. Stir in the almond flour mixture until the dough is formed (low heat).

5. Scoop the dough out and knead it into sixteen portions. Roll them into seven-inch logs and tie each one into knots. Arrange them on the pan a few inches apart.

6. Prepare the butter. Whisk the butter, garlic, parmesan, parsley, and salt. Brush the butter over the knots before baking. Bake until firm to the touch and nicely browned (15-20 min.).

7. Before serving, brush with the rest of the butter.

CHAPTER 4

BAGEL SPECIALTIES

ALMOND FATHEAD BAGELS

Servings Provided: 6

Prep & Cook Time: 27-30 minutes

Macro Counts - Per Serving:

- Calories: 377

- Net Carbohydrates: 5 g

- Fat Content: 31 g

- Protein: 20 g

Essential Ingredients:

- Almond flour (1.5 cups)

- Mozzarella cheese (2.5 cups)

- Cream cheese (3 oz.)

- Eggs (2)

- Egg white (1)

- Baking powder (1 tbsp.)

- Salt (.25 tsp.)

- Flavorless oil (1 tsp.)

- *Optional:* Everything Bagel Seasoning (*see below*)

Homemade Everything But The Bagel Seasoning:

- Black sesame seeds (1.5 tsp.)

- White sesame seeds (2 tsp.)

- Dried minced onion (1 tsp.)

- Poppy seeds (.5 tsp.)

- Dried minced garlic (1 tsp.)

- Sea salt (1 tsp.)

- *Optional*: Sesame seeds

Preparation Technique:

1. Set the oven at 400° F/204° C. Mix the bagel seasoning and set it aside.

2. Prepare a baking tray with a layer of parchment baking paper.

3. Toss both types of cheese into a microwave-safe container. Set the microwave timer for one minute and set it aside.

4. Whisk the almond flour, salt, and baking powder in a mixing container. Whisk and add in one of the eggs. Shred the mozzarella and fold in with the cream cheese.

5.   Portion the dough into six balls. Poke your finger in the center and work it to shape the bagels. Place the bagels on the baking tray.

6.   Whisk the egg white with a little water and gently brush the tops. Leave plain or add your favorite toppings. Bake for 12 to 15 minutes. Brown the tops to your liking.

7.   Serve with a portion of grass-fed butter.

8.   *Note:* As the cheese cools, it may become more challenging to mix. You can microwave the dough for ten seconds to make it more pliable.

ASIAGO BAGELS

Servings Provided: 8

Prep & Cook Time: 30 minutes

Macro Counts - Per Serving:

- Calories: 293

- Net Carbohydrates: 6 g

- Fat Content: 21 g

- Protein: 20 g

Essential Ingredients:

- Shredded mozzarella (2 cups)

- Shredded asiago (1 cup)

- Cream cheese (.25 cup)

- Free-range eggs (2)

- Organic almond flour (1.5 cups)

- Gluten-free baking powder (1 tbsp.)

- Sea salt (.5 tsp.)

Preparation Technique:

1. Program the oven temperature setting to 400° F/204° C.

2. Combine the almond flour, eggs, salt, and baking powder.

3. In a microwave-safe container, melt the mozzarella and cream cheese. Combine the melted mixture, almond flour mixture, and ¾ cup of shredded asiago.

4. Shape into a ball and knead until each of the fixings is thoroughly combined. Break the dough into eight pieces and shape each into a ball. Shape them into bagel forms.

5. Sprinkle the remaining ¼ cup of asiago cheese onto the bagels. Arrange on a baking pan and bake for about 20 minutes.

CAULIFLOWER EVERYTHING BAGELS

Servings Provided: 2

Prep & Cook Time: 38-40 minutes

Macro Counts - Per Serving:

- Calories: 185

- Net Carbohydrates: 6 g

- Fat Content: 11 g

- Protein: 11 g

Essential Ingredients:

- Cauliflower florets (6 cups)

- Shredded sharp cheddar cheese (1 cup)

- Large egg (1)

- Everything Bagel Seasoning (2.5 tsp.)

Preparation Technique:

1. Set the oven temperature at 425° F/218° C. Cover a baking tin using a layer of parchment paper.

2. Finely chop the cauliflower in a food processor. Dump it into a microwave-safe dish.

3. Cover the dish loosely with plastic wrap. Microwave using the high-heat setting for three minutes and wait for it to cool slightly.

4. Wrap the cauliflower in a kitchen tea towel to remove the moisture. Toss it into the bowl and stir in the egg and cheddar cheese.

5. Divide the dough into eight portions on the baking sheet. Flatten and shape the bagels. Sprinkle with seasoning.

6. Bake for 22-25 minutes.

7. Prepare in advance if desired.

CHEESY KETO BAGELS

Servings Provided: 6

Prep & Cook Time: 17 minutes

Macro Counts - Per Serving:

- Calories: 356

- Net Carbohydrates: 5.9 g

- Fat Content: 27.9 g

- Protein: 22.8 g

Essential Ingredients:

- Almond flour (1.5 cups)

- Coconut flour (3 tbsp.)

- Baking soda (1 tsp.)

- Cream of tartar (2 tsp.)

- Shredded mozzarella (2.5 cups)

- Cream cheese (2 oz.)

- Large eggs (3)

- Sesame seeds (2 tsp.)

Preparation Technique:

1. Warm the oven to reach 400° F/204° C.

2. Prepare a baking sheet with a layer of paper.

3. Sift the coconut flour, almond flour, cream of tartar, and baking soda.

4. Add the shredded mozzarella and cream cheese to a safe dish and microwave for 90 seconds. Remove the container from the microwave and stir. Return and cook for one more minute until they're thoroughly combined.

5. In another small mixing bowl, whisk two eggs. Add the whisked eggs in with the dry ingredients.

6. Add the melted cheese mixture into the bowl of flour and eggs.

7. With your hands, knead the dough until all ingredients are completely incorporated with one another.

8. Divide the dough into six portions.

9. Gently roll each of the portions into a log shape and attach the two ends to make the log into the bagel circle. Arrange the dough on the paper-lined baking sheet.

10. Whisk the remaining egg and gently brush the egg wash over the tops. Sprinkle the sesame seeds.

11. Bake the bagels until golden brown or for approximately 15 to 17 minutes. Watch them closely when you hit the 15-minute marker.

12. Move the pan of bagels from the oven. Be sure to cool for at least 15 minutes for the best results.

13. Once they are cool, just store in a closed container.

COCONUT FATHEAD BAGELS

Servings Provided: 2

Prep & Cook Time: 25-30 minutes

Macro Counts - Per Serving:

- Calories: 234

- Net Carbohydrates: 4 g

- Fat Content: 16 g

- Protein: 14 g

Essential Ingredients:

- Coconut flour (.5 cup)

- Aluminum-free baking powder (2 tbsp.)

- Cream cheese (2 oz.)

- Shredded mozzarella cheese (2.5 cups)

- Melted butter (2 tbsp.)

Preparation Technique:

1. Set the oven temperature setting to 400° F/204° C.

2. Cover a baking tray using a piece of parchment baking paper.

3. Sift the baking powder and coconut flour into a container.

4. Melt the mozzarella and cream cheese for one minute using high-power in the microwave. Stir and cook for another minute.

5. Mix in whisked eggs, butter, and coconut flour mixture to form the dough into six pieces. Roll and shape the bagel.

6. Place the bagels on the baking tin. Bake until lightly browned (approx. 12-16 min.). Serve.

COCONUT FLOUR GARLIC BAGELS

Servings Provided: 6

Prep & Cook Time: 40 minutes

Macro Counts - Per Serving:

- Calories: 191

- Net Carbohydrates: 3 g

- Fat Content: 16 g

- Protein: 8 g

Essential Ingredients:

- Melted butter (.33 cup)

- Sifted coconut flour (.5 cup)

- Baking powder (.5 tsp.)

- Eggs (6)

- Salt (.5 tsp.)

- Garlic powder (1.5 tsp.)

- *Optional*: Guar gum or xanthan gum (2 tsp.)

- *Also Needed*: Donut pan

Preparation Technique:

1. Set the oven at 400° F/204° C.

2. Spritz the pan with a mist of cooking oil.

3. Blend the salt, eggs, garlic powder, and butter.

4. Whisk the flour with the baking powder and xanthan gum.

5. Mix it all into a batter until it is lump-free.

6. Scoop into the pan. Bake for 15 minutes. Cool for 10-15 minutes.

7. Transfer the bagels from the pan to cool or serve. Store in the fridge.

Croissant Bagels

Servings Provided: 7

Prep & Cook Time: 35-40 minutes

Macro Counts - Per Serving:

- Calories: 83

- Net Carbohydrates: 1.1 g

- Fat Content: 0.7 g

- Protein: 3.4 g

Essential Ingredients:

- Eggs (3)
- Cream of tartar (.25 tsp.)
- Softened cream cheese (2 tbsp.)
- Melted butter (2 tbsp.)
- Sifted coconut flour (2 tbsp.)
- Sweetener of choice - Erythritol (1.5 tsp.) or Liquid stevia (15 drops)
- Cream of tartar (.25 tsp.) + Baking soda (.5 tsp.) mixed
- Sea salt (.125 tsp.)
- Also Needed: Donut/bagel pan

Preparation Technique:

1.   Set the oven temperature to 300° F/149 ° C.

2.   Lightly spritz the pan with cooking oil spray.

3.   Separate the egg whites from the yolks.

4.   Add the cream of tartar with the egg whites. Combine until stiff peaks form. Set the container to the side for now.

5.   Whisk the egg yolks in a separate mixing container. Combine the mixture with the melted butter, cream cheese, baking soda, cream of tartar mixture, coconut flour, sea salt, and sweetener of choice. Continue beating until the egg yolk mixture is thoroughly incorporated.

6.   Gently fold in (do not whisk) the egg yolk mixture into the egg white mixture until incorporated. Scoop into the pan.

7.   Set a timer to bake the bagels for 20 to 25 minutes. Once it's done, remove and cool.

French Toast Gluten-Free Bagels

Servings Provided: 6

Prep & Cook Time: 25 minutes

Macro Counts - Per Serving:

- Calories: 207

- Net Carbohydrates: 3 g

- Fat Content: 16 g

- Protein: 8 g

Essential Ingredients:

- Melted butter (.33 cup)

- Eggs (6)

- Cinnamon (1 tbsp.)

- Sugar-free vanilla extract (2 tsp.)

- Maple extract (1 tsp.)

- Stevia glycerite (5-10 drops or Swerve sweetener (1-1.5 tbsp.)

- Baking powder (.5 tsp.)

- Salt (.5 tsp.)

- Sifted coconut flour (.5 cup)

- *Optional:* Xanthan gum or guar gum (.5 tsp.)

Preparation Technique:

1. Warm the oven to 400° F/204° C.

2. Lightly grease a six-count muffin pan.

3. Blend the eggs with the cinnamon, stevia, salt, vanilla extract, maple extract, and butter in a large mixing container.

4. Whisk the coconut flour with the baking powder and guar/xanthan gum in a medium mixing bowl.

5. Combine everything and spoon into the pan and bake for 15 minutes.

MOZZARELLA DOUGH BAGELS

Servings Provided: 6

Prep & Cook Time: 25 minutes

Macro Counts - Per Serving:

- Calories: 203

- Net Carbohydrates: 2.4 g

- Fat Content: 16.8 g

- Protein: 16.8 g

Essential Ingredients:

- Mozzarella cheese (1.75 cups)

- Salt (1 pinch)

- Almond meal (.75 cup)

- Baking powder (1 tsp.)

- Full-fat cream cheese (2 tbsp.)

- Egg (1 medium)

Preparation Technique:

1.   Set the oven temperature at 425° F/220° C.

2.   Combine the shredded mozzarella with the cream cheese and almond meal in a mixing container. Melt it in the microwave for one minute.

3.   Stir the mixture and continue using the high-setting for another 30 seconds.

4.   Whisk the egg, baking powder, salt, and any other flavorings.

5.   Portion the dough into six segments. Roll into balls and then into cylinder shapes.

6.   Securely fold the ends together to form the bagels, so they do not become separated during the cooking process.

7.   Arrange the bagels on the baking pan and sprinkle with a few of the sesame seeds.

8.   Bake until golden brown (about 15 min.).

ONION - GLUTEN-FREE BAGELS

Servings Provided: 6

Prep & Cook Time: 45 minutes

Macro Counts - Per Serving:

- Calories: 78

- Net Carbohydrates: 1 g

- Fat Content: 45 g

- Protein: 5 g

Essential Ingredients:

- Flaxseed meal (3 tbsp.)

- Coconut flour (2 tbsp.)

- Baking powder (.5 tbsp.)

- Eggs (4 - separated)

- Dried minced onion (1 tsp.)

Preparation Technique:

1. Set the oven temperature to reach 325° F/163° C.

2. Lightly spray a six-count donut pan with a spritz of cooking oil.

3. Combine the baking powder with the flaxseed meal, coconut flour, and onion in a medium mixing container.

4. Whisk the egg whites in a mixing container until foamy using an electric mixer. Whisk the yolks and combine the rest of the fixings.

5. Wait for about five to ten minutes for the batter to expand. Scoop it into the prepared baking tin. Garnish using more dried onion as desired.

6. Bake for ½ hour. Cool in the oven.

PIZZA BAGELS

Servings Provided: 6

Prep & Cook Time: 22-25 minutes

Macro Counts - Per Serving:

- Calories: 449

- Net Carbohydrates: 6 g

- Fat Content: 35 g

- Protein: 28 g

Essential Ingredients:

- Baking powder (1 tbsp.)

- Almond flour (2 cups)

- Garlic powder (1 tsp.)

- Onion powder (1 tsp.)

- Dried Italian seasoning (1 tsp.)

- Large eggs (2)

- Shredded mozzarella cheese - low moisture (3 cups)

- Cream cheese (3 tbsp.)

- Low-carb pizza sauce (.25 cup)

- Chopped pepperoni slices (2.5 oz.)

- Dried oregano (1 tsp.)

- Shredded parmesan cheese (2 tbsp.)

Preparation Technique:

1.   Warm the oven in advance at 425° F/218° C.

2.   Cover a rimmed baking tin with a layer of parchment baking paper.

3.   Sift the almond flour, garlic powder, baking powder, dried Italian seasoning, and onion powder.

4.   In a microwave-safe container, mix the mozzarella and cream cheese. Cook for

5.   1 ½ minutes. Remove from the microwave and stir to combine. Continue heating at 30-second increments as needed.

6.   In a mixing bowl, whisk and add the eggs and flour mixture, stirring until all of the fixings are well combined.

7.   Once everything is well combined, mix in the pepperoni to the dough. Little by little, add and mix in the sauce. The dough will be relatively soft.

8.   Divide the dough into six portions, rolling into a ball.

9.   Prepare rings and stretch to make a bagel. Top each one with oregano and parmesan.

10. Bake on the middle rack until golden brown (12-14 min.).

POPPY - SESAME SEED BAGELS

Servings Provided: 6

Prep & Cook Time: 30-35 minutes

Macro Counts - Per Serving:

- Calories: 350

- Net Carbohydrates: 5 g

- Fat Content: 29 g

- Protein: 20 g

Essential Ingredients:

- Baking powder (1 tsp.)

- Almond flour (1.5 cups)

- Mozzarella cheese - shredded (2.5 cups)

- Sesame cheese (8 tsp.)

- Poppy seeds (8 tsp.)

- Large eggs (2)

Preparation Technique:

1.   Set the oven temperature to 400° F/204° C.

2.   Prepare a cookie tin using a layer of parchment baking paper. Combine the almond flour and baking powder.

3.   Melt the mozzarella in a micro-safe dish for one minute.

4.   Stir and cook for one additional minute.

5.   Whisk the eggs and add the cheese mixture. Stir and combine with the rest of the fixings.

6.   Once the dough is formed, break it apart into six pieces.

7.   Stretch the dough and join the ends to form the bagels. Arrange on the baking sheet.

8.   Sprinkle with the seed combination and bake for 15 minutes.

ROSEMARY BAGELS

Servings Provided: 4

Prep & Cook Time: 1 hour 10 minutes

Macro Counts - Per Serving:

- Calories: 285

- Net Carbohydrates: 4.5 g

- Fat Content: 23 g

- Protein: 13 g

Essential Ingredients:

- Salt (.25 tsp.)

- Psyllium husk powder (3 tbsp.)

- Almond flour (1.5 cups)

- Baking soda (.75 tsp.)

- Xanthan gum (.75 tsp.)

- Whole egg (1)

- Egg whites (3)

- Warm water (.5 cup)

- Freshly chopped rosemary (1 tbsp.)

- Avocado oil (as needed)

Preparation Technique:

1. Set the oven temperature at 350° F/177° C.

2. Spritz a bagel mold with avocado oil.

3. Whisk the xanthan gum, almond flour, baking soda, and salt together in a mixing container.

4. In another dish, whisk the eggs and warm water. Stir in the psyllium husk.

5. Add the liquid fixings to dry ingredients.

6. Press the dough into the mold. Sprinkle rosemary on top.

7. Bake for 45 minutes. Pop it out and cool for 15 minutes before slicing.

CHAPTER 5

MUFFIN SPECIALTIES

APPLE & ALMOND MUFFINS

Servings Provided: 12

Prep & Cook Time: 25 minutes

Macro Counts - Per Serving:

- Calories: 184

- Net Carbohydrates: 10 g

- Fat Content: 15 g

- Protein: 5 g

Essential Ingredients:

- Almond flour (2.5 cups)

- Cinnamon (1 tsp.)

- Eggs (2)

- Maple syrup (4 tbsp.)

- Melted butter (.33 cup)

- Thinly sliced apple (1)

- Also Needed: 12-cup muffin tin with paper holders

Preparation Technique:

1. Heat the oven to reach 350° F/177° C.

2. Mix all of the fixings except for the apple.

3. Peel and fold in the apple slices. Scoop the dough mix to the cups.

4. Set a timer to bake the muffins for 15 minutes. Thoroughly cool the muffins before storage.

5. Keep them in the refrigerator for the best results.

BACON & CHEESE CAULIFLOWER MUFFINS

Servings Provided: 6 @ 2 each

Prep & Cook Time: 45 minutes

Macro Counts - Per Serving:

- Calories: 110

- Net Carbohydrates: 2.4 g

- Fat Content: 8 g

- Protein: 7 g

Essential Ingredients:

- Cauliflower rice (3 cups)

- Cheddar cheese - shredded (1 cup)

- Baking powder (1 tsp.)
- Almond flour (.25 cup)
- Oregano (1 tbsp.)
- Chopped bacon (7 slices)
- Garlic powder (1 tbsp.)
- Parsley (1 tbsp.)
- Black pepper and salt (as desired)
- Paprika (1 tbsp.)
- Large eggs (2)
- Crumbled feta (.25 cup)
- Suggested: 12-count muffin tin

Preparation Technique:

1. Set the oven temperature to reach 350° F/177° C.

2. Prepare the riced cauliflower. It is essential to use a heavy container when processing the riced cauliflower.

3. Cook, drain, and chop the bacon.

4. Fold in each of the dry fixings with the bacon and cheese. Whisk and add the eggs and mix well.

5. Prepare the muffin tin with baking cups. Add the mixture to each one and top with the feta cheese.

6. Bake for 35 minutes and serve.

BLUEBERRY MUFFINS

Servings Provided: 12

Prep & Cook Time: 37 minutes

Macro Counts - Per Serving:

- Calories: 247

- Net Carbohydrates: 4 g

- Fat Content: 21.5 g

- Protein: 7.5 g

Essential Ingredients:

- Swerve - sugar replacement - granular (.5 cup)

- Almond flour (3 cups)

- Coarse kosher salt (.25 tsp.)

- Bak. powder (1.5 tsp.)

- Eggs (3 large)

- Coconut oil (.33 cup)

- Vanilla extract (.5 tsp.)

- Almond milk (.33 cup)

- Whole blueberries (1 cup)

- *Also Suggested*: 12-count muffin tin

Preparation Technique:

1. Set the oven temperature setting at 350° F/177° C.

2. Prepare the muffin pan with 12 paper liners.

3. Sift/whisk the almond flour with the sweetener, salt, and baking powder into a large mixing container.

4. Mix in the coconut oil until the mixture has small pieces of coconut oil running through it. Work in the eggs, milk, and vanilla extract.

5. Slowly, fold in the blueberries.

6. Scoop the mixture into the prepared baking cups.

7. Set the timer for 25 minutes and bake until the tops are golden.

8. Test using a toothpick or other cake tester. If it comes out clean, they're ready.

CHOCOLATE MUFFINS

Servings Provided: 8

Prep & Cook Time: 40 minutes

Macro Counts - Per Serving:

- Calories: 111

- Net Carbohydrates: 3 g

- Fat Content: 10 g

- Protein: 3 g

Essential Ingredients:

- Melted cacao butter (4.6 oz./9 tbsp.)

- Chopped steamed pumpkin/organic canned pumpkin (2 cups)

- Coconut oil (.5 cup)

- Collagen protein powder (.5 cup)

- Eggs (3)

- Coconut flour (.5 cup)

- Cacao powder (1 cup)

- Vanilla extract (3 tsp.)

- Apple cider vinegar (2 tsp.)

- Salt (1 pinch)

- Granulated sugar-free sweetener ex. monk fruit/erythritol blend (4 tbsp.)

- Baking soda (1 tsp.)

Preparation Technique:

1. Heat the oven to reach 350° F/177° C.

2. Add each of the fixings into a blender (omit the collagen). Mix until thoroughly combined. Lastly, toss in the collagen and blend using the lowest speed setting until just incorporated.

3. Grease or line the muffin tins. Spoon the protein muffin mix into the pan.

4. Set a timer and bake for ½ hour, checking at the 25-minute marker.

5. Cool slightly before removing the muffins from the pan.

6. Serve with berries and coconut cream or right out of the pan.

CINNAMON ORANGE GLUTEN-FREE MUFFINS

Servings Provided: 12

Prep & Cook Time: ½ hour

Macro Counts - Per Serving:

- Calories: 243

- Net Carbohydrates: 2 g

- Fat Content: 22 g

- Protein: 7 g

Essential Ingredients:

- Almond flour (3 cups)

- Ghee or coconut oil - melted - but not hot (.5 cup)

- Eggs (4 large)

- Cinnamon (3 tbsp.)

- Baking soda (1 tsp.)

- Cloves (.25 tsp.)

- Nutmeg (1 tsp.)

- Orange zest (3 tbsp.)

- Lemon juice (1 tsp.)

- Stevia or another Keto-friendly sweetener (as desired)
  Also Needed:

- Metal or silicone muffin tin

- Cake tester

Preparation Technique:

1. Set the oven at 350° F/177° C before baking time.

2. Prepare a metal muffin pan using a spritz of cooking oil.

3. Whisk each of the fixings in a medium mixing bowl and dump them into the pan.

4. Bake for 18-20 minutes. Serve when ready.

CORNBREAD MUFFINS

Servings Provided: 6

Prep & Cook Time: ½ hour

Macro Counts - Per Serving:

- Calories: 191

- Net Carbohydrates: 2 g

- Fat Content: 17 g

- Protein: 6 g

Essential Ingredients:

- Almond flour (.75 cup)

- Coconut flour (.25 cup)

- Baking powder (2 tsp.)

- Salt (1 tsp.)

- Ghee (2 tbsp.)

- Eggs (3)

- Coconut milk (.5 cup)

Preparation Technique:

1. Set the oven temperature at 350° F/177° C. Lightly grease a 6-count muffin tin using a spritz of coconut oil or muffin liners.

2. Combine all of the fixings and mix well in a large bowl.

3. Dump the batter into the muffin pan.

4. Set the timer for the cornbread to bake for 20 minutes.

CREAM CHEESE BLUEBERRY MUFFINS

Servings Provided: 12

Prep & Cook Time: ½ hour

Macro Counts - Per Serving:

- Calories: 155

- Net Carbohydrates: 2 g

- Fat Content: 14 g

- Protein: 3 g

Essential Ingredients:

- Unchilled cream cheese (16 oz.)

- Low-carb sweetener of choice (.5 cup)

- Eggs (2)

- Xanthan gum optional (.25 tsp.)

- Sugar-free vanilla extract (.5 tsp.)

- Blueberries (.25 cup)

- Sliced almonds (.25 cup)

Preparation Technique:

1. Set the oven temperature setting at 350° F/177° C.

2. Mix the cheese until it's a creamy texture.

3. Stir in the eggs, sweetener, vanilla, and xanthan gum.

4. Fold in the blueberries and almonds.

5. Scoop into the molds and bake for about 20 minutes.

6. Chill and serve.

ENGLISH MUFFIN

Servings Provided: 1

Prep & Cook Time: 25 minutes - varies

Macro Counts - Per Serving:

- Calories: 200

- Net Carbohydrates: 2.5 g

- Fat Content: 12 g

- Protein: 8 g

Essential Ingredients:

- Melted butter or coconut oil (.5 tbsp.)

- Whisked egg (1)

- Unsweetened almond/coconut milk (1 tbsp. or Half & Half)

- Coconut flour (1 tbsp.)

- Baking powder (.5 tsp.)

- *Optional*: Vanilla extract (.125 tsp.)

- *Optional*: Liquid stevia (6 drops)

- *Optional*: Sea Salt (1 pinch)

Preparation Technique:

1.   Heat the oven to reach 400° F/204° C or use a microwave.

2.   Melt the oil or butter in a ramekin. Add the remainder of the fixings to the bowl, and quickly stir until the clumps are gone.

3.   Pop it into the microwave for 1.5 minutes or bake for 12-15 minutes.

4.   Loosen the edges and transfer them to a cutting surface. Slice in half sideways.

5.   Lightly brown on each side in a skillet prepared with oil or butter. Gently press the muffins in the pan with the spatula as they toast.

6.   Serve any way you like it, but stay Keto!

LEMON BLACKBERRY MUFFINS

Servings Provided: 12

Prep & Cook Time: 40-45 minutes

Macro Counts - Per Serving:

- Calories: 277

- Net Carbohydrates: 5 g

- Fat Content: 25 g

- Protein: 8 g

Essential Ingredients:

- Almond flour (2 cups)

- Sea salt (.125 tsp.)

- GF aluminum-free baking powder (2 tsp.)

- Coconut flour (1 tbsp.)

- Heavy cream (.5 cup)

- Unchilled large eggs (2)

- Melted butter (.25 cup)

- Lemon juice (1 tbsp.) & zest (1 lemon)

- Pure vanilla extract (1 tsp.)

- Liquid stevia (12 drops)

- Fresh firm blackberries or cherries - fresh or frozen (1.5 cups)

- Chopped pecans (.5 cup)

Preparation Technique:

1.   Set the oven temperature to reach 350° F/177° C.

2.   Prepare a muffin pan with paper liners.

3.   Measure and add the baking powder, almond flour, and salt into a food processor.

4.   Pour in the butter, cream, eggs, lemon juice, lemon zest, vanilla, and stevia. Blend until creamy.

5.   Fold in the blackberries and pecans. Empty the mixture into the muffin tins.

6.   Bake the muffins for 30-35 minutes. Cool in the tins before removing.

7.   *Notes*: If you do not have a food processor, use an electric mixer.

8.   If you are using frozen berries, do not defrost before adding to the recipe.

PEPPERONI PIZZA GLUTEN-FREE MUFFINS

Servings Provided: 12

Prep & Cook Time: 40 minutes

Macro Counts - Per Serving:

- Calories: 182

- Net Carbohydrates: 2 g

- Fat Content: 14 g

- Protein: 8 g

Essential Ingredients:

- Cream cheese (5 oz.)

- Asiago cheese shredded (.5 cup)

- Coconut flour (.25 cup)

- Baking powder (1 tsp.)

- Almond flour (.66 cup)

- Salt (.5 tsp.)

- Water (3 tsp.)

- Eggs (5)

- Mini pepperonis (.5 cup/about 2 oz.)

- Mozzarella cheese - shredded & divided (1 cup)

Preparation Technique:

1. Program the oven before the baking time to reach 400° F/204° C.

2. Spritz the muffin molds with cooking oil spray.

3.   Whisk the eggs with the cream cheese, salt, grated Asiago cheese, both types of flour, baking powder, and water.

4.   Fold in ½ cup of the mozzarella and the pepperoni.

5.   Fill the muffin cups about half-full and toss in the rest of the mozzarella cheese.

6.   Bake until the muffins are firm and lightly browned (25-30 min.).

7.   Enjoy them hot, at room temperature, or straight from the fridge.

PISTACHIO MUFFINS

Servings Provided: 12

Prep & Cook Time: 35 minutes

Macro Counts - Per Serving:

- Calories: 198

- Net Carbohydrates: 3 g

- Fat Content: 17 g

- Protein: 6 g

Essential Ingredients:

- Almond milk - unsweetened/plain (.5 cup)

- Unsalted butter (.5 cup)

- Large brown eggs (4)

- Swerve confectioners (.25 cup)

- Large brown eggs (4)

- Organic stevia blend - ex. Pyure (.25 cup)

- Pistachio & vanilla extract (1 tsp. each)

- Blanched almond flour (1 cup)

- Organic coconut flour – gluten-free (.5 cup)

- Baking powder (2 tsp.)

- Xanthan gum (.5 tsp.)

- Himalayan Pink Salt (1 tsp.)

- Pistachio nuts crushed (.5 cup)

Preparation Technique:

1. Set the oven temperature to reach 325° F/163° C.

2. Whisk the eggs in a large mixing container.

3. In another container, melt the butter until softened. Mix in the sweetener, almond milk, and each of the extracts.

4. In a medium container, add the rest of the fixings (omit the pistachios for now).

5. Whisk, making sure there are no clumps.

6. Add the dry ingredients into a large bowl and mix well. Fold in the crushed pistachios until blended.

7. Grease 12 muffin cups or use paper liners. Pour the batter evenly into each well.

8.   Gently tap the container to release any air bubbles.

9.   Bake for 25 to 30 minutes. Before removing from the molds, be sure to let them cool first.

CHAPTER 6

HOMEMADE WAFFLES & PANCAKES

ALMOND CREAM CHEESE KETO PANCAKES

Servings Provided: 4

Prep & Cook Time: 12 minutes

Macro Counts - Per Serving:

- Calories: 203

- Net Carbohydrates: 2.3 g

- Fat Content: 15 g

- Protein: 16 g

Essential Ingredients:

- Almond flour (.5 cup + 1 tbsp.)

- Full-fat cream cheese (.5 cup)

- Eggs (4)

- Granulated sweetener (1 tsp.)

- *Optional*: Baking powder for a super-fluffy pancake (.5 tsp.)

- Butter for frying (as needed)

Preparation Technique:

1.   Mix all of the fixings in a blender.

2.   Fry the pancakes in melted butter in a large skillet using the medium-temperature setting.

3.   Once they start to bubble, flip them over. The pancakes should be small (four-inches in diameter) as a perfect toasting size.

4.   Reheat the next day if desired.

Almond Flour Pancakes

Servings Provided: 2/8 small cakes

Prep & Cook Time: 8-10 minutes

Macro Counts - Per Serving:

- Calories: 339

- Net Carbohydrates: 4 g

- Fat Content: 30 g

- Protein: 12 g

Essential Ingredients:

- Heavy whipping cream (2 oz.)

- Eggs (2 large)

- Granulated erythritol (2 tsp.)

- Finely ground almond flour (.5 cup)

- Sea salt (1 pinch)

- Bak. powder (.25 tsp.)

- Unsalted butter (1 tsp.)

Preparation Technique:

1.   Whisk the whipping cream with the egg yolks, salt, and low-carb sweetener in a large mixing container until it's smooth.

2.   Whisk the baking powder and flour into the batter.

3.   In a separate container, mix the egg whites using an electric mixer to create soft peaks. Gently mix it into the batter.

4.   Prepare a large skillet using the medium-temperature setting to melt the butter. Cook until lightly browned (3 min.), gently flip each pancake, and continue cooking for an additional two minutes.

ALMOND FLOUR - GLUTEN-FREE PUMPKIN PANCAKES

Servings Provided: 4 or 12 small pancakes

Prep & Cook Time: 20-25 minutes

Macro Counts - Per Serving:

- Calories: 89

- Net Carbohydrates: 2 g

- Fat Content: 8 g

- Protein: 3 g

Essential Ingredients:

- Almond flour (1 cup)

- Cinnamon (2 tsp.)

- Ground ginger (.5 tsp.)

- Allspice (.25 tsp.)

- Ground cloves (.125 tsp.)

- Salt (1 pinch)

- Baking powder (.5 tsp.)

- Canned pumpkin (.25 cup)

- Oil (2 tbsp.)

- Almond milk - unsweet (.25 cup)

- Erythritol (1 tbsp.)

- Stevia glycerite (.125 tsp.)

- Eggs (2)

- For the Pan: Butter or oil (as needed)

Preparation Technique:

1. Sift the baking powder, flour, spices, and salt.

2. Stir in the rest of the fixings until thoroughly combined (omit the egg whites). Whip the whites into a stiff peak, and mix into the batter.

3. Drop by heaping tablespoonfuls into a large heated skillet. Add a little butter/oil to the pan.

4. Use the medium-temperature setting, flipping each pancake once.

COCONUT FLOUR GLUTEN-FREE PANCAKES

Servings Provided: 12

Prep & Cook Time: 20 minutes

Macro Counts - Per Serving:

- Calories: 77

- Net Carbohydrates: 1 g

- Fat Content: 7 g

- Protein: 1 g

Essential Ingredients:

- Unsalted butter - melted (.25 cup)

- Eggs (3 + 1 more as needed the batter is too thick)

- Heavy cream sour cream (.25 cup)

- Stevia (1 packet)

- Coconut flour (.25 cup)

- Baking powder (.5 tsp.)

- Salt (.25 tsp. or more to taste)

- Vanilla extract (.5 tsp.)

- *Optional*: Water as needed

Preparation Technique:

1.   Whisk the butter with the cream, eggs, salt, stevia, and vanilla.

2.   In another medium container, whisk the coconut flour with the baking powder. Combine it all and let it rest to thicken (15-30 minutes).

3.   Prepare a large skillet using the medium heat setting with a spritz of cooking oil.

4.   Spoon the batter by heaping tablespoons onto the skillet to make the pancakes (2-inch in diameter).

5.   Use the spatula to flatten out the thick batter to form thinner or flatter cakes.

HEALTHY KETO WAFFLES

ALMOND FLOUR WAFFLES

Servings Provided: 8

Prep & Cook Time: 10 minutes

Macro Counts - Per Serving:

- Calories: 237

- Net Carbohydrates: 3 g

- Fat Content: 23 g

- Protein: 5 g

Essential Ingredients:

- Almond flour sifted (1 cup + more if needed)

- Bak. powder (1.5 tsp.)

- Salt (.25 tsp.)

- *Optional*: Xanthan gum (.25 tsp.)

- Heavy cream (1 cup + a little water as needed)

- Oil (2 tbsp.)

- Eggs (3)

Preparation Technique:

1.   Heat the waffle maker while you prepare the batter.

2.   Sift the flour with the baking powder, xanthan gum, and salt in a big mixing container.

3.   Whisk and add in the eggs and preferred oil.

4.   Slowly add in the heavy cream. Adjust the waffle batter texture using flour or water as needed.

5.   Add the prepared batter into the waffle maker. Wait until the waffles are nicely browned (about 5 min.). Serve as desired.

BREAKFAST PIZZA WAFFLES

Servings Provided: 2

Prep & Cook Time: 15 minutes

Macro Counts - Per Serving:

- Calories: 604

- Net Carbohydrates: 7.6 g

- Fat Content: 48 g

- Protein: 31 g

Essential Ingredients:

- Large eggs (4)

- Grated parmesan cheese (4 tbsp.)

- Baking powder (1 tsp.)

- Italian seasoning (1 tsp.)

- Psyllium husk powder (1 tbsp.)

- Almond flour (3 tbsp.)

- Salt and pepper (as desired)

- Bacon grease (1 tbsp.)

- Tomato sauce (.5 cup)

- Cheddar cheese (3 oz.)

- *Optional*: Pepperoni (14 slices)

Preparation Technique:

1.   Use an immersion blender to prepare all of the fixings together until it thickens (Omit the tomato sauce and cheese).

2.   Heat the waffle iron. Prepare the waffle batter in two batches.

3.   Pour the tomato sauce (¼ cup for each) and cheese (1.5 ounces each) onto each waffle.

4.   Broil for three to five minutes in the oven. Add pepperoni if desired but count the carbs.

COCONUT BELGIAN STYLE WAFFLES

Servings Provided: 4

Prep & Cook Time: 7-10 minutes

Macro Counts - Per Serving:

- Calories: 247

- Net Carbohydrates: 3 g

- Fat Content: 19 g

- Protein: 11 g

Essential Ingredients:

- Eggs (6)

- Melted butter or ghee (4 tbsp.)

- Salt (.5 tsp.)

- Baking powder (.5 tsp.)

- Coconut flour (.33 cup)

- *Optional:* Stevia drops (.125 tsp.)

Preparation Technique:

1. Use a blender to combine the butter and eggs until thoroughly mixed.

2.   Pour in the stevia, salt, and baking powder. Blend to combine.

3.   Fold in the flour and wait for it to thicken (5 min.)

4.   Pour in small amounts of water as needed. Prepare in the waffle maker and cook until browned to your liking to serve.

CRISPY SWEET CINNAMON KETO WAFFLES

Servings Provided: 2

Prep & Cook Time: 9-10 minutes

Macro Counts - Per Serving:

- Calories: 331

- Net Carbohydrates: 4 g

- Fat Content: 29 g

- Protein: 11 g

Essential Ingredients:

- Super-fine almond flour (.5 cup)

- Salt (.25 tsp.)

- Baking soda (.25 tsp.)

- Preferred sweetener (.5 tsp.)

- Baking powder (.25 tsp.)

- Ground cinnamon (.25 tsp.)

- Cloves (.125 tsp.)

- Nutmeg (.125 tsp.) *Wet Fixings:*

- Vanilla extract (1 tsp.)

- Butter (2 tbsp.)

- Eggs (2)

Preparation Technique:

1.   Whisk the dry fixings in a small mixing container. Set it to the side for now.

2.   Separate the eggs into two small mixing dishes.

3.   Melt the butter and mix it with the vanilla and egg yolks.

4.   Beat the egg whites to form stiff peaks when lifting the beaters.

5.   Combine the dry fixings with the egg yolks. Slowly, add the whites.

6.   Mix until smooth and pour into the preheated waffle iron.

FLUFFY CHEESE WAFFLES

Servings Provided: 4

Prep & Cook Time: 11-15 minutes

Macro Counts - Per Serving:

- Calories: 231

- Net Carbohydrates: 5 g

- Fat Content: 18 g

- Protein: 9.6 g

Essential Ingredients:

- Cream cheese (4 oz.)

- Vanilla extract (1 tsp.)

- Eggs (4)

- Melted butter (1 tbsp.)

- Bak. powder (1.5 tsp.)

- Powdered stevia (1 tbsp.)

- Coconut flour (4 tbsp.)

- *Optional:* Cinnamon or Lily's Chocolate Chips

Preparation Technique:

1. Warm the waffle iron. Spritz with a misting of cooking oil spray.

2. Combine each of the fixings in a blender and mix for one minute or until everything is smooth. Alternately, blend with an electric mixer for one to two minutes, making sure to remove all of the lumps. Add a pinch of cinnamon or chocolate chips if desired.

3. Prepare the batter using ¼ cup portions or less for smaller waffles. Prepare and serve.

KETO CHOCOLATE WAFFLES

Servings Provided: 5

Prep & Cook Time: 35-40 minutes

Macro Counts - Per Serving:

- Calories: 289

- Net Carbohydrates: 3.4 g

- Fat Content: 27 g

- Protein: 7.2 g

Essential Ingredients:

- Medium eggs (5)

- Unsweetened cocoa (.25 cups)

- Coconut flour (4 tbsp.)

- Swerve granulated sweetener (4 tbsp./as desired)

- Baking powder (1 tsp.)

- Vanilla (2 tsp.)

- Full-fat milk or cream (3 tbsp.)

- Melted salted butter (1 stick)

Preparation Technique:

1.   Whisk the egg whites for a few minutes to form stiff peaks in a small mixing container.

2.   Whisk the yolk with the coconut flour, cocoa, sweetener, and baking powder in a medium mixing container.

3.   Melt the butter and mix it with the milk and vanilla. Add it to the rest of the fixings. Fold in a spoonful of the prepared egg whites and add the batter to the preheated waffle maker.

4.   Prepare the waffles until each one is golden brown and serve.

CHAPTER 7

CRUNCHY BREADSTICKS & CRACKERS

BREADSTICK CHOICES

ALMOND COCONUT & FLAX BREADSTICKS

Servings Provided: 5 servings/20 sticks

Prep & Cook Time: 1 hour 5 minutes

Macro Counts - Per Serving:

- Calories: 334

- Net Carbohydrates: 4.2 g

- Fat Content: 27 g

- Protein: 13 g

Essential Ingredients:

- Almond flour (1 cup)

- Flax meal/ground flaxseed (.75 cup)

- Coconut flour (.25 cup)

- Salt (1 tsp.)

- Psyllium husk powder (1 tbsp.)

- Chia seeds (2 tbsp.)

- Lukewarm water (1 cup (+) 2 tbsp. if the dough is dry) *Toppings:*

- Mixed seeds - ex. Poppy/sesame/caraway seeds (4 tbsp.)

- Egg yolks (2 large - For egg-free - use water or melted ghee)

- Coarse sea salt - Pink Himalayan (1 tsp.) *Optional Garnishes:*

- Pesto

- BBQ sauce

- Marinara sauce

- Keto Cheese sauce

Preparation Technique:

1. Set the oven to 360° F/182° C. 99

2. Combine all of the ingredients to form a dough. Work it until it holds together and set it aside for 15-20 minutes.

3. Divide the dough into four segments. Then, into five pieces. Form the stick about ten inches long.

4. Put the breadsticks on a paper-lined baking tin, and brush with the yolks or ghee.

5. Give them a sprinkle of salt, seeds, and parmesan cheese.

6. Bake for 15-20 minutes until crispy.

GARLIC & HERB BREADSTICK BITES

Servings Provided: varies - approx. 7 @ 9 sticks

Prep & Cook Time: 30-35 minutes

Macro Counts - Per Serving:

- Calories: 135.2

- Net Carbohydrates: 2.4 g

- Fat Content: 4.2 g

- Protein: 5.4 g

Essential Ingredients:

- Cheddar cheese (.25 cup - shredded)

- Unchilled cream cheese (2 oz.)

- Almond flour (.5 cup)

- Garlic (1 tsp.)

- Dried chives (1 tsp.)

- Coconut flour (1 tbsp.)

- Egg white (1)

Preparation Technique:

1. Warm the oven to reach 350° F/177° C.

2. Prepare a baking tin with a layer of paper.

3. Combine the cream cheese with the cheddar in a mixing container.

4. Mince and add in the garlic, chives, almond and coconut flour, and slightly beaten egg white. It should not be crumbly or dry, but soft.

5. Add the mixture to a plastic bag. Snip away about a 1-inch corner, or use a pastry bag to pipe the dough onto the baking pan.

6. Make 3-inch strips with the prepared dough. Flatten each one with the tongs of a fork.

7. Bake for 10 to 15 minutes. Serve.

ITALIAN BREADSTICKS

Servings Provided: 16

Prep & Cook Time: 30-35 minutes

Macro Counts - Per Serving:

- Calories: 130

- Net Carbohydrates: 2 g

- Fat Content: 10 g

- Protein: 8 g

Essential Ingredients:

- Garlic (2 cloves)

- Almond flour (1.5 cups)

- Nutritional yeast (1 tbsp.)

- Baking powder (2 tsp.)

- Dried parsley (2 tsp.)

- Psyllium husk powder (1 tbsp.)

- Dried basil (.5 tsp.)

- Shredded mozzarella cheese (2.5 cups)

- Cream cheese (3 oz.)

- Garlic salt (1 tsp.)

- Eggs (2)

- Grated parmesan cheese (2 tbsp.)

- Flavorless oil - as needed for prep

- Olive oil for brushing the tops

Preparation Technique:

1. Warm the oven at 400° F/204° C. Cover a baking sheet with parchment paper.

2. Prepare the garlic cloves with a press.

3. Place the mozzarella and cream cheese into the bowl and cook for one minute.

4. Add and whisk the almond flour with the nutritional yeast, psyllium husk powder, parsley, basil, oregano, garlic salt, and baking powder in another bowl.

5. Add the eggs in with the mozzarella cheese, fresh garlic, and cream cheese.

6. Combine and mix in the parmesan, then add in the dry fixings.

7. Divide the dough into eight pieces, shaping them into 16 logs/breadsticks.

8. Arrange them on a layer of parchment baking paper and place them on the top oven rack.

9. Bake for 12 minutes. Rotate the breadsticks about halfway through the baking cycle to ensure it's cooking evenly.

10. When the time is up, transfer to the countertop and lightly brush olive oil over the tops. Pop it back into the oven to bake for an additional three minutes.

11. Cool slightly before serving.

KETO BREAD TWISTS

Servings Provided: 10

Prep & Cook Time: ½ hour

Macro Counts - Per Serving:

- Calories: 204

- Net Carbohydrates: 1 g

- Fat Content: 18 g

- Protein: 7 g

Essential Ingredients:

- Almond flour (.5 cup)

- Coconut flour (4 tbsp.)

- Salt (.5 tsp.)

- Baking powder (1 tsp.)

- Shredded cheese - mozzarella suggested (1.5 cups)

- Butter (2.33 oz.)

- Egg (2 - Use 1 for brushing the tops)

- Green pesto (2 oz.)

Preparation Technique:

1. Set the oven temperature ahead of baking time to reach 350° F/177° C. Prepare a baking tray with a layer of baking paper.

2. Whisk all the dry fixings.

3. Use the low-temperature setting to melt the butter and cheese together. Stir until smooth and mix in the egg. Combine all of the fixings to make the dough.

4. Roll the dough between two layers of baking paper until it is about one inch thick. Remove the top sheet.

5. Spread the pesto on top of the dough and slice into one-inch strips.

6. Twist the dough and place on the baking tin. Brush the twists with the second egg (whisked first).

7. Bake until golden brown (15-20 min.).

TASTY CRACKERS

ALMOND FLAXSEED CRACKERS

Servings Provided: 40 crackers/10 per serving

Prep & Cook Time: 35-40 minutes

Macro Counts - Per Serving:

- Calories: 173

- Net Carbohydrates: 3 g

- Fat Content: 15 g

- Protein: 6 g

Essential Ingredients:

- Almond flour (1 cup)
- Ground flaxseed (1 tbsp.)
- Water (3 tbsp.)

- Fine-grain sea salt (.5 tsp.)

- *Optional:* Flaked sea salt

Preparation Technique:

1. Heat the oven in advance to reach 350° F/177° C.

2. Prepare the dough by combining the first four fixings. Lay it out on a sheet of parchment paper and cover with a second sheet. Flatten the dough - either with a rolling pin your hands, but press the dough into a 1/8-inch thickness.

3. Sprinkle with the flaked sea salt. Use a pizza slicer to make the cuts about ½- to 1-inch sections with a triangular cut.

4. Arrange them on a paper-lined baking tray. Set a timer for the crackers and bake (20 to 25 min.).

5. Thoroughly cool to store.

BUTTER CRACKERS

Servings Provided: 25

Prep & Cook Time: 35 minutes

Macro Counts - Per Serving:

- Calories: 90

- Net Carbohydrates: 1 g

- Fat Content: 8 g

- Protein: 2 g

Essential Ingredients:

- Egg whites (2)

- Softened - not melted – salted butter (8 tbsp.)

- Almond flour (2.25 cups)

- Salt (1 pinch)

Preparation Technique:

1. Set the oven temperature to 350° F/177° C.

2. Combine the egg whites and butter in a mixing container using the low-medium setting using a hand mixer until smooth.

3. Fold in the salt and almond flour – mixing at low speed until well mixed.

4. Place the dough between 2 sheets of parchment and roll out on the baking tin.

5. Score the crackers lightly using a pizza cutter or sharp knife into approximately 1.5-inch squares.

6. Pop the tray into the oven to bake (10-15 min.). Transfer them to the countertop until slightly cooled. Gently break the crackers apart on the scored lines.

7. They will last up to one week at room temperature. If stored in the fridge, the crackers could lose some of the crunchiness.

BUTTERY PESTO CRACKERS

Servings Provided: 6

Prep & Cook Time: 25-30 minutes

Macro Counts - Per Serving:

- Calories: 205

- Net Carbohydrates: 3 g

- Fat Content: 19 g

- Protein: 5 g

Essential Ingredients:

- Garlic (1 pressed clove)

- Ground black pepper (.25 tsp.)

- Salt (.5 tsp.)

- Almond flour (1.25 cups)

- Baking powder (.5 tsp.)

- Dried basil (.25 tsp.)

- Cayenne pepper (1 pinch)

- Basil pesto (2 tbsp.)

- Butter (3 tbsp.)

Preparation Technique:

1. Warm up the oven to reach 325° F/163° C.

2. Prepare a baking tray using a sheet of parchment baking paper.

3. Hand press or mince the garlic.

4. Whisk the baking powder, salt, flour, and pepper.

5. Toss in the cayenne, garlic, and basil. Stir in the pesto and form a dough mixture.

6. Fold in the butter with your fingers or a fork until a dough ball is formed.

7. Arrange on the baking sheet and spread it out until thin.

8. Bake for 14 to 17 minutes. Remove from the oven, cool thoroughly, and cut into crackers.

CHIA SEED CRACKERS

Servings Provided: 36

Prep & Cook Time: 1.5 hours

Macro Counts - Per Serving:

- Calories: 28

- Net Carbohydrates: 0.28 g

- Fat Content: 2.15 g

- Protein: 0.88 g

Essential Ingredients:

- Ground chia seeds (.5 cup)

- Shredded cheddar cheese (3 oz.)

- Ice water (1.25 cups)

- Psyllium husk powder (2 tbsp.)

- Olive oil (2 tbsp.)

- *Spices Needed* - 0.25 tsp. of each:

- Xanthan gum

- Onion powder

- Oregano

- Paprika

- Salt

- Pepper

- Garlic powder

- Also Needed: Spice grinder

Preparation Technique:

1. Use a spice grinder to prepare the chia seeds and add to the rest of the dry fixings.

2. Set the oven setting to reach 375° F/191° C.

3. Blend the oil into the dry components to make a sandy consistency. Add the water into the mixture to form the dough.

4. Fold in the cheddar and mix well. Place on a Silpat to rest five minutes or so. Roll out the dough until it's thin.

5. Bake for 30-35 minutes. Remove and slice into individual crackers.

6. Place back in the oven to broil for five to seven minutes until crispy.

7. Chill and serve or store.

FATHEAD CRACKERS

Servings Provided: 6

Prep & Cook Time: 20 minutes

Macro Counts - Per Serving:

- Calories: 203

- Net Carbohydrates: 3 g

- Fat Content: 17 g

- Protein: 11 g

Essential Ingredients:

- Almond flour/meal (.75 cup)

- Shredded mozzarella/Edam cheese (1.75 cups)

- Cream cheese (2 tbsp.)

- Egg (1)

- *Optional*: Flavorings of choice (.5 tsp.)

- Salt (as desired)

Preparation Technique:

1. Line a baking tray with parchment paper.

2. Combine and melt both types of cheese, and the flour in a microwaveable bowl using the high setting for one minute. Stir well and cook for ½ minute.

3. Whisk the egg, salt, and seasonings. Mix gently.

4. Roll the dough until thin and cut into small squares. Arrange on a paper-lined baking pan.

5. Bake the crackers at 425° F/218° C until crispy or for five minutes per side.

6. Cool and store in the fridge.

GOAT CHEESE CRACKERS

Servings Provided: 12

Prep & Cook Time: 30 minutes

Macro Counts - Per Serving:

- Calories: 99

- Net Carbohydrates: 2 g

- Fat Content: 8 g

- Protein: 3 g

Essential Ingredients:

- Baking powder (1 tsp.)

- Fresh rosemary (2 tbsp.)

- Butter (4 tbsp.)

- Coconut flour (.5 cup)

- Goat cheese (6 oz.)

Preparation Technique:

1. Set the oven temperature to 380° F/194° C.

2. Use a food processor to mix all of the fixings, processing until creamy smooth.

3. Roll the dough out using a rolling pin until it's about ¼ to ½-inches thick.

4. Use a cookie cutter or knife to portion the crackers.

5. Place them on a paper-lined pan. Pop them into the oven to bake for 15-20 minutes.

HEMP HEART CRACKERS

Servings Provided: 36

Prep & Cook Time: 1 hour 10 minutes

Macro Counts - Per Serving:

- Calories: 76

- Net Carbohydrates: 1 g

- Fat Content: 6 g

- Protein: 1 g

Essential Ingredients:

- Almond flour (1 cup)

- Coconut flour (.5 cup + more as needed)

- Hemp hearts (.5 cup)

- Baking powder (3 tsp.)

- Optional: Xanthan gum (1 tsp.)

- Salt for topping (.5 tsp.)

- Baking soda (.25 tsp.)

- Salted butter – very cold (6 tbsp.)

- Melted butter with salt (4 tbsp.)

- Olive oil (2 tbsp.)

- Ice water (.66 cup)

Preparation Technique:

1. Preheat the oven to 400° F/204° C.

2. Toss the hemp hearts, both types of flour, baking soda, baking powder, and salt in a mixing container – mixing well.

3. Grate the chilled butter, mixing it into the flour mixture.

4. Stir in the olive oil and stir until it's blended. Add the water.

5. Pop the dough into the fridge for at least 30 minutes.

6. At that time, dust a Silpat or sheet of parchment paper with coconut flour.

7. Prepare the dough (¼-inch thickness), and dust with flour. Cut into the desired shapes.

8. Poke tiny holes in the crackers using a toothpick. Bake them for 15 to 20 minutes.

9. Prepare the butter with ½ tsp. of salt to brush the crackers while they're hot. For best results, turn off the oven. For a crispy cracker, put the pan in the oven to bake for five minutes longer.

10. Remove and cool the batch entirely before storing them.

SPICY CHILI CRACKERS

Servings Provided: 30 crackers

Prep & Cook Time: 1 hour 15 minutes

Macro Counts - Per Serving:

- Calories: 37

- Net Carbohydrates: 0.7 g

- Fat Content: 3.1 g

- Protein: 1 g

Essential Ingredients:

- Paprika (.5 tsp.)

- Cumin (.5 tsp.)

- Chili pepper spice (1.5 tsp.)

- Onion powder (1 tsp.)

- Almond flour (.75 cup)

- Coconut flour (.25 cup)

- Salt (.5 tsp.)

- Egg (1 whole)

- Unsalted butter (.25 cup)

Preparation Technique:

1. Warm the oven at 350° F/177° C.

2. Prepare a baking tray with a layer of parchment paper.

3. Toss all of the fixings into a food processor and pulse the mixture into dough.

4. Portion the dough into two parts and place one of them on the paper. Cover with another layer of paper. Flatten it using a rolling pin.

5. Slice the sheet into crackers and continue with the second ball.

6. Arrange them on the tray and bake for eight to ten minutes.

7. Transfer to the countertop to slightly cool and enjoy.

TOASTED SESAME CRACKERS

Servings Provided: 6

Prep & Cook Time: 30 minutes

Macro Counts - Per Serving:

- Calories: 213

- Net Carbohydrates: 3 g

- Fat Content: 17 g

- Protein: 11 g

Essential Ingredients:

- Grated Asiago cheese (.5 cup)

- Egg white (1)

- Dijon mustard (1 tbsp.)

- Toasted sesame seeds (.25 cup)

- Almond flour (1 cup)

- Paprika (1 tsp.)

- Salt (.5 tsp.)

Preparation Technique:

1. Heat the oven until it reaches 325° F/163° C.

2. Lightly grease a sheet of foil in a baking pan.

3. Combine all of the fixings except for the salt into a processor. Pulse until it shapes into dough. Take it from the processor and roll out the dough to form a log about 1.5-inch round before slicing them into ¼-inch slices.

4. Arrange the crackers on the baking sheet and sprinkle with the salt. Bake them for 17 to 20 minutes.

CHAPTER 8

FLATBREAD & PIZZA SPECIALTIES

Pizza Crust

ALMOND FLOUR PIZZA CRUST

Servings Provided: 8

Prep & Cook Time: 55 minutes

Macro Counts - Per Serving:

- Calories: 182

- Net Carbohydrates: 3 g

- Fat Content: 14 g

- Protein: 8 g

Essential Ingredients:

- Almond flour (1.5 cups)

- Baking powder (.5 tsp.)

- Grated parmesan cheese (.5 cup)

- Flax meal or Whole psyllium husks (1 tbsp.)

- Basil (.5 tsp.)

- Garlic powder (.5 tsp.)

- Oregano (.5 tsp.)

- Large eggs (2)

- Water (2 tbsp. or more if needed)

- Olive oil (1 tbsp.)

Preparation Technique:

1. Warm the oven at 375° F/191° C.

2. Whisk the almond flour with the parmesan cheese, basil, oregano, psyllium baking powder, and garlic powder.

3. In another dish, whisk the oil with the water and eggs. Pour the mixture into the dry fixings, adding more water as needed.

4. Shape the dough into a ball. Prepare it between two layers of parchment baking paper. Roll the dough out and transfer it to a pizza pan. Discard the top piece of paper.

5. Bake until the crust is browned for about 20-25 minutes. Cool for about 15 minutes.

6. Flip the crust over in the pan. Discard the bottom paper.

7. Add the pizza sauce and chosen toppings as desired.

8. Bake under the oven broiler to melt the cheese and fixings to your liking. After you switch over to the broil

setting, watch the pizza closely, so the toppings do not burn.

EGGLESS & CHEESELESS KETO PIZZA CRUST

Servings Provided: 8

Prep & Cook Time: 40 minutes

Macro Counts - Per Serving:

- Calories: 209

- Net Carbohydrates: 2.8 g

- Fat Content: 17 g

- Protein: 13 g

Essential Ingredients:

- Almond flour (2 cups)

- Baking powder (2 tsp.)

- Whey protein isolate or casein (1.25 cups)

- Xanthan gum (1 tsp.)

- Water (.75 cup + 2 tsp.)

- Olive oil (.25 cup)

- Salt

- Toppings (to your liking)

Preparation Technique:

1. Whisk the protein powder with the almond flour, xanthan gum, salt, and baking powder.

2. Mix in the oil and warm water to create the dough.

3. Arrange the dough on a piece of parchment baking paper and using wet hands - make it flat and pizza shaped. (*Note*: Don't roll with a rolling pin. It will stick to the parchment paper.)

4. Bake for ten minutes at 350° F/177° C.

5. Transfer the crust to the countertop to add the desired toppings. Bake until the crust is nicely browned (15-20 min.).

GARLIC FOCACCIA

Servings Provided: 8

Prep & Cook Time: 40 minutes

Macro Counts - Per Serving:

- Calories: 245

- Net Carbohydrates: 3.4 g

- Fat Content: 19 g

- Protein: 10.2 g

Essential Ingredients:

- Almond flour (1 cup)

- Salt (2 pinches)

- Bak. powder (1 tsp.)

- Ground flaxseed (1 cup)

- Eggs (6)

- Olive oil (.25 cup)

- Minced cloves of garlic (2)

- Dried oregano & basil (1 tsp. each)

- Also Needed: 8x8-inch glass baking dish

Preparation Technique:

1. Heat the oven to reach 350° F/177° C.

2. Line a baking dish with a sheet of baking paper.

3. Sift or whisk the flour in with the spices, baking powder, and flaxseed into a mixing container.

4. One by one, add the eggs and garlic, whisking as you go.

5. Add the oil and combine the batter. Oil your hands before preparing the dough, and add the batter.

6. Bake for 25 minutes and serve, or cool to store. You can keep them on the countertop or freeze for later use.

7. When it's time to eat, wrap the focaccia in a damp paper towel. Prepare in the microwave for 10-15 seconds.

THIN CRUST WHITE PIZZA

Servings Provided: 4

Prep & Cook Time: 30 minutes

Macro Counts - Per Serving:

- Calories: 352

- Net Carbohydrates: 4.6 g

- Fat Content: 29 g

- Protein: 20 g

Essential Ingredients:

The Crust:

- Unflavored egg white protein powder (.25 cup)

- Almond flour (.5 cup)

- Grated parmesan cheese (.5 cup)

- Pink Himalayan salt (.25 tsp.)

- Large egg (1) *The Topping:*

- Cream cheese (2 tbsp.)

- Onion or garlic powder (1 tsp.)

- Hard goat cheese - your choice (.5 cup)

- Heavy whipping cream (1 tbsp.)

- Crumbled feta cheese (.33 cup)

- Small red onion (1)

- Seedless Kalamata olives (.25 cup)

- Olive oil (1 tbsp.)

Preparation Technique:

1. Set the oven temperature to reach 400° F/204° C.

2. Prepare an iron skillet or baking tin with a layer of baking paper.

3. Whisk the dry fixings in a mixing bowl. Mix in the egg by hand. Dump the batter into the baking tray, spreading evenly. Bake the batter for 10-15 minutes.

4. Prepare the white sauce by mixing the onion or garlic powder, cream cheese, and cream. Mix well.

5. Peel the skin off of the onion and slice. Grate the hard cheese and crumble the feta. Chop the olives.

6. Remove the crust when browned and add the white sauce, both types of cheese, olives, and onion.

7. Bake for another ten minutes. Remove and slice into quarters. Top with some lettuce leaves with a drizzle of olive oil and serve.

TOPPED PIZZA

CHEESE & ALMOND PIZZA

Servings Provided: 4

Prep & Cook Time: 20-25 minutes

Macro Counts - Per Serving:

- Calories: 450

- Net Carbohydrates: 5 g

- Fat Content: 45 g

- Protein: 15 g

Essential Ingredients:

- Eggs (2)

- Alfredo sauce (.5 cup)

- Cheddar cheese (4 oz.)

- Butter (5 tbsp.)

- Almond meal (1 cup)

- Stevia (1.5 tsp.)

- Garlic powder (.5 tsp.)

- Baking powder (1.5 tsp.)

- Thyme (.25 tsp.)

- Oregano (.5 tsp.)

Preparation Technique:

1. Spritz a pizza baking pan using a cooking oil spray. Set the oven at 350° F/177° C.

2. Combine the dry fixings and fold in the eggs. Melt and add the butter to the mixture.

3. Prepare the crust and spread it out evenly onto the pan. Cook the crust for five to seven minutes. Transfer it from the oven and add the alfredo sauce.

4. Garnish it with the cheese. Bake for another five to seven minutes.

5. Serve when it's browned to your liking.

PEPPERONI PIZZA

Servings Provided: 6

Prep & Cook Time: 25-30 minutes

Macro Counts - Per Serving:

- Calories: 335

- Net Carbohydrates: 3.2 g

- Fat Content: 27 g

- Protein: 18 g

Essential Ingredients:

The Base:

- Mozzarella cheese (2 cups/8 oz.)

- Almond flour (.75 cup)

- Psyllium husk powder (1 tbsp.)

- Cream cheese (3 tbsp./1.5 oz.)

- Large egg (1)

- Italian seasoning (1 tbsp.)

- Pepper & salt (.5 tsp. each) *The Toppings:*

- Mozzarella cheese (1 cup or 4 oz.)

- Rao's Tomato Sauce (.5 cup)

- Pepperoni (16 slices)

- *Optional*: Sprinkle of oregano

Preparation Technique:

1. Warm the oven at 400° F/204° C.

2. Microwave the mozzarella cheese until completely melted. Add all other base fixings (omitting the olive oil) and mix well.

3. Knead the dough into a ball and spread it out into a circle.

4. Bake the crust for ten minutes. Flip it and bake for two to four additional minutes.

5. Toss the crust with the toppings of your choice and bake for another three to five minutes.

6. Cool slightly, slice, and serve.

FLATBREAD

CHEESY KETO FLATBREAD

Servings Provided: 6

Prep & Cook Time: 20-25 minutes

Macro Counts - Per Serving:

- Calories: 161

- Net Carbohydrates: 1.3 g

- Fat Content: 14 g

- Protein: 8 g

Essential Ingredients:

- Olive oil (.5 tbsp.)

- Almond flour (6 tbsp.)

- Grated mozzarella (.75 cup)

- Spicy spaghetti seasoning (2 tsp.)

- Grated cheddar cheese (.5 cup)

- Sea salt (1 pinch)

- Cubed cream cheese (2 tbsp.)

- Egg (1)

Preparation Technique:

1. Set the oven temperature at 400° F/204° C.

2. Spritz oil on a layer of parchment baking paper to fit the baking tray.

3. Whisk the spaghetti seasoning with the mozzarella, flour, and sea salt.

4. Toss in the cubed cream cheese.

5. Set the microwave timer for 45 seconds. Stir and microwave on high for another 20 seconds. Stir and fold in the egg.

6. Scoop the dough onto the tray and shape it into a rectangle. Toss the cheddar cheese over the stretched dough.

7. Bake until the bread is a nice golden brown and the cheese has melted (15-18 min.).

8. Use a sharp knife and slice into six servings.

SPICY SPAGHETTI SEASONING

Servings Provided: 53 teaspoons

Prep & Cook Time: 5 minutes

Macro Counts - Per Serving - *Per Teaspoon:

- Calories: 4.1

- Net Carbohydrates: 1.2 g

- Protein: 0.2 g

Essential Ingredients:

Dried Spices:

- Dehydrated minced onion (3 tbsp.)

- Red pepper flakes (1 tbsp.)

- Parsley (2 tbsp.)

- Thyme (1 tbsp.)

- Basil (3 tbsp.)

- Oregano (2 tbsp.)

- Onion powder (1 tbsp.)

- Freshly cracked black pepper (1 tbsp.)

- Garlic powder (2 tbsp.)

- Sea salt (1 tbsp.)

- Powdered monk fruit/erythritol sweetener or white sugar (1 tbsp.)

Preparation Technique:

1. Measure out each ingredient and add to a medium-sized bowl.

2. Whisk to combine.

3. Store in an airtight container such as a glass jar or zipper-type bag, and store in the pantry for up to six months.

GARLIC & BASIL FLATBREAD

Servings Provided: 8

Prep & Cook Time: 25 minutes

Macro Counts - Per Serving:

- Calories: 56

- Net Carbohydrates: 0.6 g

- Fat Content: 4.5 g

- Protein: 3.6 g

Essential Ingredients:

- Mozzarella cheese (.75 cup)

- Cream cheese (1 tbsp.)

- Egg (1)

- Almond flour (2 tbsp.)

- Garlic powder (1 tbsp.)

- Basil (1 tsp.)

Preparation Technique:

1. Warm the oven ahead of baking time to 350° F/177° C.

2. Melt both of the cheese items and mix in the almond flour and egg.

3. Flatten the mixture onto a parchment paper-lined baking tin.

4. Garnish using garlic to bake for 20 minutes.

GARLIC FATHEAD DOUGH FLATBREAD

Servings Provided: 8

Prep & Cook Time: 27 minutes

Macro Counts - Per Serving:

- Calories: 192

- Net Carbohydrates: 2.6 g

- Fat Content: 15 g

- Protein: 9 g

Essential Ingredients:

The Dough:

- Coconut flour (.33 cup)

- Swerve Confectioners (1 tbsp.)

- Baking powder (.5 tsp.)

- Salt (.25 tsp.)

- Shredded mozzarella cheese -part-skim - low-moisture (1.5 cups)

- Cream cheese (2 tbsp.)

- Large eggs (2)

- Heavy whipping cream (2 tbsp.) *The Topping:*

- Butter - melted (3 tbsp.)

- Garlic powder (1 tsp.)

- Salt (.5 tsp.)

- Onion powder (.5 tsp.)

- Grated parmesan cheese (.5 cup)

Preparation Technique:

1. Set the oven temperature setting at 425° F/218° C.

2. Prepare a large baking tray using a layer of parchment baking paper.

3. Whisk the salt with the coconut flour, swerve, and baking powder in a large mixing container.

4. In a small microwave-safe container, mix the mozzarella and cream cheese. Set the timer for 45 seconds using the high setting. Remove and stir.

5. Microwave for another 45 seconds. Remove and stir again.

6. Whisk the eggs, whipping cream, and flour mixture in a medium bowl. Combine all of the fixings.

7. Arrange it on the baking tin, rolling it into a rectangle of about a 1/3-inch thickness.

8. Set a timer for seven minutes. Transfer to the countertop and prepare the topping.

9. Combine the melted butter, salt, garlic powder, and onion powder. Brush the bread and dust using the parmesan cheese.

10. Set the timer and bake for four to five minutes to your liking.

11. Cool for a few minutes and slice into eight pieces.

12. Garnish as you like with cheese and melt using the oven broiler.

INDIAN CUISINE NAAN BREAD

Servings Provided: 6

Prep & Cook Time: 17 minutes

Macro Counts - Per Serving:

- Calories: 91

- Net Carbohydrates: 3.6 g

- Fat Content: 6.4 g

- Protein: 3.5 g

Essential Ingredients:

Dry Ingredients:

- Coconut flour (.75 cup)

- Psyllium husk powder (2 tbsp.)

- Xanthan gum (1 tsp.)

- Salt (1 generous pinch)

- Bak. powder (1 tsp.)

- Sesame seeds (1 tbsp.) *Wet Ingredients:*

- Hot water (1 cup)

- Full-fat natural yogurt (.25 cup)

- Coconut oil/olive oil melted (2 tbsp.) *The Topping:*

- Coconut oil / butter / olive oil melted (2 tbsp.)

- Chopped parsley or coriander/cilantro (handful)

- Salt (1 generous pinch)

Preparation Technique:

1. Set the oven temperature to reach 356° F/180° C.

2. Combine the dry fixings in a large mixing container - removing all of the lumps.

3. Mix in the wet components and work into a dough ball.

4. Wait for a few minutes and divide the dough into six pieces. Roll them out between two sheets of parchment paper into long flatbreads. Place on an upturned baking sheet and remove the top parchment. Garnish using sesame seeds.

5. Bake 12-15 minutes until they are the way you like them. Garnish as desired.

JEWISH MATZO FLATBREAD

Servings Provided: 6

Prep & Cook Time: 8-11 minutes

Macro Counts - Per Serving:

- Calories: 28

- Net Carbohydrates: 1 g

- Fat Content: 2.2 g

- Protein: 1 g

Essential Ingredients:

- Water (.5 cup)

- Sifted almond flour (1 cup)

- Salt (1 pinch)

Preparation Technique:

1. Set the oven ahead of cooking time at 475° F/246° C.

2. Sift the flour into a mixing container. Mix in water (1 tbsp. at a time). Sprinkle in the salt and knead. Divide into four balls.

3. Prepare a baking tray and add the rolled balls of dough. Flatten into disks and pierce each one to prevent rising.

4. Bake the bread for two minutes per side. Serve as desired.

MEDITERRANEAN KETO FLATBREAD

Servings Provided: 6

Prep & Cook Time: 25 minutes

Macro Counts - Per Serving:

- Calories: 149

- Net Carbohydrates: 2 g

- Fat Content: 12 g

- Protein: 5 g

ESSENTIAL INGREDIENTS:

- Coconut flour (.5 cup)

- Ground psyllium husk powder (1 tbsp.)

- Olive oil (.25 cup)

- Boiling water (1 cup)

- Parmesan or Mozzarella cheese (.33 cup grated)

- Sea salt (.5 tsp.)

- Granulated garlic (.25 tsp.)

- Black peppercorns (.5 tsp.)

- Dried rosemary (.5 tbsp.)

Preparation Technique:

1. Set the oven temperature setting at 350° F/177° C.

2. Prepare a big baking tray with a sheet of parchment baking paper.

3. Whisk the dry fixings in a large mixing container, and add the cheese and oil.

4. Pour in hot water last, stirring as it's added. Continue stirring until the psyllium fiber and coconut flour have absorbed all of the water.

5. Flatten the dough onto the baking sheet, pressing until it's thin (less than 1/8-inch thick).

6. Bake for 20-25 minutes. When browned, place on a cooling rack, and discard the parchment paper. Cool.

7. Use a pizza cutter to slice the flatbread into squares for sandwiches.

NUTRITIONAL YEAST KETO FLATBREAD

Servings Provided: 6

Prep & Cook Time: 25 minutes

Macro Counts - Per Serving:

- Calories: 217

- Net Carbohydrates: 4 g

- Fat Content: 12 g

- Protein: 11 g

Essential Ingredients:

- Unsweetened almond milk (.5 cup)

- Nutritional yeast flakes or Dried instant yeast (1 tbsp.)

- Coconut flour (1.25 cups)

- Almond flour (1 cup)

- Garlic powder (1 tbsp.)

- Baking powder (2 tsp.)

- Italian seasoning (1 tsp.)

- Freshly cracked black pepper and salt (1 dash of each)

- Eggs (2 egg whites + 1 whole)

Preparation Technique:

1. Warm the oven to reach 320° F/160° C.

2. Warm the milk in a large microwave for 45 seconds.

3. Whisk in the active dried yeast. Cool slightly.

4. In another medium container, whisk the Italian seasoning with the salt, pepper, baking powder, coconut flour, almond flour, and garlic powder.

5. Whisk in all of the eggs.

6. Mix the wet fixings into the flour mixture, and shape it into the dough.

7. Divide it into six pieces and shape each one into a ball. Press into a flat oval shape (approximately ½ inch thick).

8. Set a timer and bake for 12-15 minutes.

QUICK & EASY FLATBREAD

Servings Provided: 6

Prep & Cook Time: 25-30 minutes

Macro Counts - Per Serving:

- Calories: 70

- Net Carbohydrates: 1.8 g

- Fat Content: 6.6 g

- Protein: 2 g

Essential Ingredients:

- Butter (1 tbsp.)

- Salt (1 pinch)

- Sifted almond flour (8 tbsp.)

- Water (1 cup)

Preparation Technique:

1. Program the oven temperature at 350° F/177° C.

2. Prep a baking tray with a layer of parchment baking paper.

3. Sift the flour with the salt. Cut in the butter.

4. Add a cup of water to the pan. Pour in the water and knead the dough. Wait for about 15 minutes.

5. Flatten the dough, making several flatbreads.

6. Bake for 15 minutes and flip over the bread and bake for another five minutes.

7. Remove from the pan and serve.

ROSEMARY & GARLIC FATHEAD FLATBREAD

Servings Provided: 4

Prep & Cook Time: 25 minutes

Macro Counts - Per Serving:

- Calories: 183

- Net Carbohydrates: 2.2 g

- Fat Content: 15 g

- Protein: 9 g

Essential Ingredients:

- Mozzarella cheese (1 cup)

- Cream cheese (1 tbsp.)

- Egg (1)

- Coconut flour (2 tbsp.)

- Butter (2 tbsp.)

- Rosemary (.5 teaspoon)

- Crushed garlic (2 cloves)

- *Also Needed*: 8 by 6-inch pan

Preparation Technique:

1. Heat the oven to reach 400° F/204° C.

2. Start by melting both types of cheese in the small dish to microwave for 1 minute.

3. Mix it well and add the coconut flour and eggs.

4. Spread it out on an oiled cookie sheet. Press it into the cookie sheet.

5. Brush a mixture of garlic, butter, and rosemary.

6. Set a timer and bake for about 15 minutes. Cool for

Vegan Coconut Flour Flatbread

Servings Provided: 6

Prep & Cook Time: 15 minutes

Macro Counts - Per Serving:

- Calories: 66

- Net Carbohydrates: 2.6 g

- Fat Content: 3.3 g

- Protein: 2 g

Essential Ingredients:

- Psyllium husk (2 tbsp.)

- Fresh coconut flour fine (.5 cup)

- Olive oil (1 tbsp.)

- Luke-warm water (1 cup)

- Baking soda (.25 tsp.)

- Olive oil to rub/oil the pan (1 tsp.)

- *Optional:* Salt (.25 tsp.)

Preparation Technique:

1. Sift and combine the psyllium husk and lump-free coconut flour into a medium mixing container.

2. Add in the tap water (105° F/41° C), olive oil, and baking soda. Stir well and knead the dough. Add salt and knead for 1 minute. Set aside for ten minutes in the mixing bowl.

3. Portion the dough into six even pieces, and roll into balls.

4. Place each of the dough balls between two pieces of parchment paper, and flatten using a rolling pin.

5. Remove the first layer of parchment paper from the bread and use a lid of a pan to cut out the round flatbread.

6. Warm a pan using the med-high-temperature setting. Lightly oil the pan using one teaspoon of oil.

7. Arrange the flatbread in the heated pan and remove the paper.

8.   Cook for two to three minutes. Flip it to the second side and continue cooking for another minute or two. Cool on a platter.

9.   Drizzle a bit of olive oil, a sprinkle of crushed garlic, and a dusting of the herbs before serving.

10.   Repeat the process with the next three flatbreads.

11.   Enjoy as a sandwich bread or right out of the pan.

CHAPTER 9

SWEET BREAD SPECIALTIES

BANANA BREAD

Servings Provided: 16

Prep & Cook Time: 1 hour 25 minutes

Macro Counts - Per Serving:

- Calories: 165

- Net Carbohydrates: 8 g

- Fat Content: 15 g

- Protein: 4 g

Essential Ingredients:

- Medium banana (1)

- Almond flour (.75 cup)

- Coconut flour (.33 cup)

- Bak. powder (1 tsp.)

- Stevia (.25 tsp.)

- Salt (.5 tsp.)

- Xanthan gum (.5 tsp.)

- Vanilla extract (1 tsp.)

- Medium eggs (6)

- Erythritol (.5 cup)

- Coconut oil (3 tbsp.)

- Melted butter (.5 cup)

Preparation Technique:

1. Heat the oven in advance to reach 325° F/163° C.

2. Grease a loaf pan.

3. Sift/whisk the almond flour with the coconut flour, xanthan gum, stevia, salt, erythritol, and baking powder.

4. Slice the banana and toss it into a food processor with the butter, oil, eggs, and vanilla extract. Pulse for one minute and combine with the rest of the fixings. Pulse for one additional minute until well blended.

5. Empty into the pan.

6. Bake for 1 ¼ hours. Serve when the urge strikes.

BLUEBERRY ENGLISH MUFFIN BREAD LOAF

Servings Provided: 12

Prep & Cook Time: 1 hour 50 minutes

Macro Counts - Per Serving:

- Calories: 156

- Net Carbohydrates: 3 g

- Fat Content: 13 g

- Protein: 5 g

Essential Ingredients:

- Butter ghee or coconut oil (.25 cup)

- Almond butter - cashew or peanut butter (.5 cup)

- Salt (.5 tsp.)

- Baking powder (2 tsp.)

- Almond flour (.5 cup)

- Almond milk unsweetened (.5 cup)

- Eggs (5)

- Blueberries (.5 cup)

Preparation Technique:

1. Program the oven temperature at 350° F/177° C.

2. Prepare a loaf pan with a layer of parchment baking paper. Lightly grease the parchment paper.

3. In the microwave, melt the nut butter and butter for ½ minute in a microwave-safe container. Stir until combined well.

4.   Sift the flour with the baking powder and salt in a mixing container. Add the nut butter mixture into the large bowl and stir to combine.

5.   Whisk/beat the eggs and almond milk. Pour into the bowl and stir well.

6.   Drop-in fresh blueberries or break apart frozen blueberries and mix them in. Gently stir into the prepared batter.

7.   Scoop the batter into the loaf pan. Set a timer to bake the loaf for 45 minutes.

8.   Transfer it to the countertop to cool for about half of an hour before removing from the pan. Test for doneness with a cake tester. When it is clean after being inserted in the center, it is done.

9.   Slice and enjoy as toast at any time.

CINNAMON SWEET ROLLS

Servings Provided: 12 rolls

Prep & Cook Time: 35 minutes

Macro Counts - Per Serving:

- Calories: 244

- Net Carbohydrates: 2 g

- Fat Content: 21 g

- Protein: 11 g

Essential Ingredients:

- Mozzarella (3 cups - shredded)

- Cream cheese (4 tbsp.)

- Almond flour (1.5 cups)

- Unchilled eggs (2)

- Baking powder (1 tsp.) *The Filling:*

- Butter (4 tbsp. - melted)

- Erythritol - powdered (4 tbsp.)

- Cinnamon (4 tsp./to
  taste) *The Icing:*

- Unchilled cream cheese (4 tbsp.)

- Greek yogurt (2 tbsp.)

- Powdered erythritol (4 tsp.)

Preparation Technique:

1. Warm the oven to reach 350° F/177° C.

2. Measure and combine the cream cheese with the mozzarella into a microwave-safe container. Heat it using 30-second intervals and mix during each pause until they thoroughly combine. Do *not* scald.

3. Whisk and mix in the egg.

4. Sift/whisk the dry components in a small mixing container until combined.

5. Mix in the dry components to the cheese and egg mixture while stirring. Use oiled hands to knead and get a uniform ball of dough. Roll the dough between two sheets of parchment to get a rectangle approximately ¼ to ½ inches thick.

6. Prepare the cinnamon filling by melting the butter with the sweetener and cinnamon. Spread the cinnamon paste over the flattened rectangle.

7. Roll it up and slice into 12 even-sized pieces.

8. Place the rolls onto an oiled non-stick baking sheet to bake for about 20 minutes.

9. Make the frosting by mixing the cream cheese with the yogurt and erythritol.

10. Spread over the warm rolls and serve. (Cool a bit before handling, or they will fall apart.

CHOCOLATE CROISSANTS

Servings Provided: 6

Prep & Cook Time: 30 minutes

Macro Counts - Per Serving:

- Calories: 218

- Net Carbohydrates: 3 g

- Fat Content: 18 g

- Protein: 10 g

Essential Ingredients:

- Cream cheese (2 tbsp.)

- Shredded mozzarella (1.5 cups)

- Egg (1)

- Low-carb sweetener - ex. Lakanto (2 tbsp.)

- Almond flour (.75 cup)

- Lily's Original Dark Chocolate (1.5 oz.)

Preparation Technique:

1.   Heat the oven to reach 350° F/177° C. Prep a baking tray with a silicone mat.

2.   Measure and add the mozzarella and cream cheese into a microwaveable bowl.

3.   Set the timer for one minute. Stir and cook for another ½ minute.

4.   Whisk and mix in the egg with the flour and sweetener.

5.   Cool the dough slightly, then knead until smooth, adding flour as needed.

6. Portion the dough into six balls and flatten them in your hand. Add two chocolate pieces in the middle.

7. Fold the dough to close and arrange them on the tray.

8. Bake them for 14 to 20 minutes. Slightly cool the croissants in the pan for about five minutes before serving.

GINGERBREAD - SLOW-COOKED

Servings Provided: 10

Prep & Cook Time: Varies - 3 hours

Macro Counts - Per Serving:

- Calories: 223
- Net Carbohydrates: 8.6 g
- Fat Content: 25 g
- Protein: 9 g

Essential Ingredients:

- Swerve sweetener (.75 cup)
- Ground ginger (1.5 tbsp.)
- Dark cocoa powder (1 tbsp.)
- Ground cinnamon (.5 tsp.)
- Baking powder (2 tsp.)
- Almond/sunflower seed flour (2.25 cups)
- Coconut flour (2 tbsp.)

- Salt (.25 tsp.)

- Ground cloves (.5 tsp.)

- Large eggs (4)

- Melted butter (.5 cup)

- Vanilla extract (1 tsp.)

- Water or almond milk (.66 cup)

- Lemon juice - fresh (1 tbsp.)

- Suggested Size Cooker: 6-quarts

Preparation Technique:

1. Spritz the cooker with cooking oil spray.

2. Sift or whisk all of the flour with the salt, cloves, baking powder, cinnamon, ginger, sweetener, and cocoa powder in a large mixing container.

3. Blend in the eggs, almond milk/water, vanilla extract, melted butter, and lemon juice.

4. Empty the batter into the slow cooker and simmer until set (2.5 to 3 hours).

5. Garnish as desired, but count the carbs.

HOT CROSS BUNS

Servings Provided: 8

Prep & Cook Time: 45 minutes

Macro Counts - Per Serving:

- Calories: 84

- Net Carbohydrates: 2.1 g

- Fat Content: 3.1 g

- Protein: 5.6 g

Essential Ingredients:

- Pumpkin spice (.5 tsp.)

- Cinnamon (.5 tsp.)

- Ground cloves (.5 tsp.)

- Coconut flour (.33 cup)

- Salt (.5 tsp.)

- Baking powder (1 tsp.)

- Psyllium husks (.33 cup)

- Swerve granulated sweetener (2 tbsp. or more to taste)

- Eggs (4 medium)

- Boiling water (1 cup

- Raisins/cacao nibs/chocolate chips

- Powdered sweetener icing mix

Preparation Technique:

1. Mix each of the dry fixings in a mixing container. Fold in the eggs.

2. Mix in the boiling water, stirring until it is evenly combined.

3. Roll it into eight balls. Add it to a baking pan.

4. Bake them in a fan-assisted oven for 20-30 minutes (350° F/177° C).

5. Prepare the icing. Mark each hot cross bun with a cross (+) using a keto-friendly powdered sweetener confectioners/icing mix and water paste mixture.

LEMON & BLUEBERRY BREAD

Servings Provided: 10

Prep & Cook Time: 60 minutes + 2 hours cooling time

Macro Counts - Per Serving:

- Calories: 207

- Net Carbohydrates: 5 g

- Fat Content: 17 g

- Protein: 9 g

Essential Ingredients:

- Almond flour (2 cups)

- Salt (.25 tsp.)

- Cream of tartar (1 tsp.)

- Coconut flour (.25 cups)

- Baking soda (.5 tsp.)

- Stevia (.75 cups)

- Blueberries (1 cup)

- Lemon zested (1)

- Vanilla extract (.5 tsp.)

- Lemon extract (1 tbsp.)

- Dairy-free mayonnaise (3 tbsp.)

- Medium egg whites (2)

- Whole large eggs (6)

PREPARATION TECHNIQUE:

1.   Heat the oven to reach 350° F/177° C.

2.   Prepare the bread pan with a layer of parchment baking paper.

3.   Whisk or sift the almond flour, salt, baking soda, stevia, and coconut flour.

4.   Fold in the egg whites, whole eggs, mayo, lemon zest, and the lemon and vanilla extract. Combine thoroughly using an electric mixer.

5.   Stir in half of the berries (.5 cup) and add to the prepared pan to bake for 20 minutes.

6.　Top it off with the remainder of the berries when it is through the first baking. Continue baking for another 50 minutes.

7.　Transfer to the counter to cool. It is best to let the bread cool for a minimum of about two hours. Serve it any time.

ZUCCHINI BREAD - SLOW-COOKED

Servings Provided: 12

Prep & Cook Time: 3 hours

Macro Counts - Per Serving:

- Calories: 174

- Net Carbohydrates: 13.8 g

- Fat Content: 16 g

- Protein: 5 g

Essential Ingredients:

- Almond flour (1 cup)

- Cinnamon (2 tsp.)

- Coconut flour (.33 cup)

- Baking powder (1.5 tsp.)

- Optional: xanthan gum (.5 tsp.)

- Salt (.5 tsp.)

- Baking soda (.5 tsp.)

- Softened coconut oil or butter (.33 cup)

- Eggs (3)

- Vanilla (2 tsp.)

- Pyure all-purpose (.5 cup)

- Shredded zucchini

- Chopped pecans or walnuts (.5 cup)

- Also Needed: 4 by 8-inch silicone bread pan

Preparation Technique:

1.   Combine the coconut and almond flour with the salt, baking soda, and powder, cinnamon, and xanthan gum. Set aside for now.

2.   Mix the oil, eggs, vanilla, and sugar in another dish. Combine the fixings.

3.   Blend in the nuts and shredded zucchini. Scoop the batter into the prepared bread pan.

4.   Arrange the cooker on the top rack (or on crunched up aluminum foil balls). You want it at least 1/2-inch from the bottom of the slow cooker.

5.   Put the top on the cooker and prepare for three hours using the high-temperature setting.

6.   Cool, wrap in foil, and place in the fridge. It is best when refrigerated.

CHAPTER 10

BAR COOKIE SPECIALTIES

BAR COOKIES

ALMOND PUMPKIN SEED BARS

Servings Provided: 8

Prep & Cook Time: **20** minutes + 2 hours chill time

Macro Counts - Per Serving:

- Calories: 262

- Net Carbohydrates: 3.8 g

- Fat Content: 25 g

- Protein: 5 g

Essential Ingredients:

- Almond flour (1 cup)

- Melted butter – divided (.25 cup)

- Erythritol – divided (.25 cup)

- Salt (.5 tsp.)

- Almond butter (.25 cup)

- Heavy cream (.25 cup)

- Cinnamon (.5 tsp.)

- Maple extract (1 tsp.)

- Xanthan gum (.25 tsp.)

- Toasted pumpkin seeds (.5 cup)

- Also Needed: 8 by 8-inch baking pan

Preparation Technique:

1. Set the oven temperature to 400° F/204° C.

2. Prepare a baking pan with a layer of parchment paper.

3. Combine 1/4 cup of the butter, salt, almond flour, and 1 tablespoon of the erythritol. Mix well.

4. Press the crust (above) into the baking pan or dish. Bake for 12-15 minutes. Transfer to the countertop and let it cool.

5. Use a blender to combine the almond butter, rest of the melted butter, xanthan gum, maple extract, cinnamon, and heavy cream. Blend until smooth and creamy. Scoop it into the prepared crust and top with the toasted pumpkin seeds.

6. Store in the fridge for a minimum of two hours; overnight is best.

7. Slice into eight squares.

CHIA SEED BAR COOKIES

Servings Provided: 14

Prep & Cook Time: 15-20 minutes

Macro Counts - Per Serving:

- Calories: 121

- Net Carbohydrates: 1.5 g

- Fat Content: 11 g

- Protein: 2.5g

Essential Ingredients:

- Toasted almonds (.5 cup)

- Coconut oil - divided (1 tbsp.) + (1 tsp.)

- Erythritol - divided (4 tbsp.)

- Butter (2 tbsp.)

- Heavy cream (.25 tsp.)

- Liquid stevia (.25 tsp.)

- Vanilla extract (1.5 tsp.)

- Unsweetened and shredded coconut flakes (.5 cup)

- Chia seeds (.25 cup)

- Coconut cream (.5 cup)

- Coconut flour (2 tbsp.)

- Also Needed: Food Processor

Preparation Technique:

1.   Add the toasted almonds into the food processor and pulse until crumbly.

2.   Toss in one tablespoon of the coconut oil and two tablespoons of the erythritol. Continue processing until you have almond butter. (Now you have another new usable product.)

3.   Heat a pan and melt the butter. Mix in the heavy cream, erythritol, stevia, and vanilla. Stir until they're bubbly and fold in the almond butter. Stir to blend.

4.   In a blender, grind the chia seeds to make a powdery mix.

5.   In another pan, toast the coconut flakes and mix with the chia seeds.

6.   Melt the coconut cream in a separate skillet.

7.   Now, combine all of the fixings and add the melted coconut cream, flour, and coconut oil. Store in the refrigerator for one hour.

8.   When it's ready, slice into squares and serve.

CHOCOLATE CHIP KETO BARS

Servings Provided: 12

Prep & Cook Time: ½ hour

Macro Counts - Per Serving:

- Calories: 190

- Net Carbohydrates: 3 g

- Fat Content: 17 g

- Protein: 7 g

Essential Ingredients:

- Blanched almond flour (1.75 cups)

- Coconut flour (1 tbsp.)

- Baking powder (1 tsp.)

- Salt (.25 tsp.)

- Sugar-free brown sugar (.75 cup)

- Granulated sweetener of choice monk fruit or erythritol (.25 cup)

- Almond butter or any smooth nut or seed butter (.5 cup)

- Coconut oil - softened (2 tbsp.)

- Eggs (unchilled - 2 large)

- Vanilla extract (1/8 tsp.)

- Keto chocolate chips (.25 to .5 cup)

Preparation Technique:

1. Warm the oven to reach 350° F/177° C.

2. Line an 8 x 8-inch pan with a layer of parchment baking paper and set aside.

3. Sift the almond flour with the coconut flour, baking powder, and salt, and mix well.

4.   In another container, whisk the sugars, butter, coconut oil, and eggs, until glossy. Stir in the vanilla extract.

5.   Slowly add the dry with the wet ingredients, and mix until just combined. Fold in the chocolate chips. Transfer to the lined pan.

6.   Bake until just golden brown on top (22-25 min.). Remove from the oven and let the cake cool in the pan completely. Slice into 12 bars.

COCONUT CHIA BARS

Servings Provided: 6

Prep & Cook Time: 1 hour

Macro Counts - Per Serving:

- Calories: 164

- Net Carbohydrates: 3.5 g

- Fat Content: 14 g

- Protein: 4 g

Essential Ingredients:

- Water (.5 cup)

- Chia seeds (4 tbsp.)

- Coconut oil (1 tbsp.)

- Confectioners Swerve (1 tbsp.)

- Vanilla extract (.25 tsp.)

- Shredded dried coconut meat – unsweetened (1 cup)

- Cashews (.5 cup)

- Also Needed: 9 by 9-inch cookie sheet

Preparation Technique:

1. Set the oven temperature to 350° F/177° C.

2. Soak the seeds 15 minutes until gel-like, and mix with the coconut, oil, swerve, and vanilla extract. Lastly, add the cashews.

3. Line the mixture, using parchment paper, onto the baking tin. Press until it is about a 3/4-inch thickness, and bake for 45 minutes.

4. Slice into six bars and enjoy!

COCONUT CREAM KETO BROWNIES

Servings Provided: 6

Prep & Cook Time: 35 minutes

Macro Counts - Per Serving:

- Calories: 175

- Net Carbohydrates: 2 g

- Fat Content: 17 g

- Protein: 3 g

Essential Ingredients:

- Raw unsweetened cocoa powder (.25 cup)

- Coconut flour (.25 cup)

- Sugar substitute (.5 cup)

- Sea salt (1 pinch)

- Melted coconut butter (.75 cup)

- Coconut cream (.33 cup)

- Pure vanilla extract (1 tsp.)

- Melted butter or coconut oil – 2 tbsp.

- Egg (1)

- Baking soda (.25 tsp.)

- Also Needed: 9 x 3-inch loaf pan

Preparation Technique:

1. Lightly spritz the pan with cooking oil spray. Set the oven temperature in advance to reach 350° F/177° C.

2. Whisk the coconut flour with the cocoa powder, sugar substitute, salt, and baking powder in a large mixing container.

3. Mix the coconut butter, butter, and coconut cream. Whisk in the vanilla and egg.

4. Fold in the dry components and mix well.

5.   Add the batter into the greased pan. Set a timer to bake until a cake tester inserted in the middle comes out clean (20 min.).

6.   Cool at room temperature. Slice into squares to serve.

TART LEMON-LIME BARS

Servings Provided: 16

Prep & Cook Time: 45-50 minutes

Macro Counts - Per Serving:

- Calories: 192

- Net Carbohydrates: 2 g

- Fat Content: 19.2 g

- Protein: 3.2 g

Essential Ingredients:

- Almond flour (1.5 cups)

- Coconut - for the crust - unsweetened & shredded (.5 cup)

- Melted butter – divided (1 cup)

- Erythritol (.25 cup)

- Freshly grated ginger (1 tbsp.)

- Lime juice (.25 cup each)

- Zest of lime (1 tbsp.)

- Lemon juice (.25 cup)

- Egg yolks (6)

- Xanthan gum (5 tsp.)

- Plain gelatin (2 tbsp.) *The Garnish*:

- Toasted shredded coconut (.25 cup)

- Chopped fresh mint (1 tbsp.)

- Also Needed: 8 by 8-inch-baking pan

Preparation Technique:

1. Cover the pan using parchment baking paper. Heat the oven temperature to reach 350° F/177° C.

2. Sift/whisk the almond flour, ginger, erythritol, ½ cup of the coconut, and ½ cup of melted butter.

3. Press the mixture into the baking dish. Bake until the crust is golden or for 10-12 minutes. Let it cool thoroughly.

4. Pour the rest of the butter into a pan using the low heat setting. Stir in the lime zest, lemon, and lime juice.

5. Crack the eggs one by one. Separate and add the egg yolks. Continue to stir until thickened.

6. Transfer from the heat and add the gelatin and xanthan gum. Stir until it dissolves. Pour over the cooked crust. Return the pan to the hot oven and bake for 15-18 minutes. The bars should be set in the center.

7.   Cool the bars slightly before you garnish with some fresh mint and toasted coconut.

8.   Slice into bars and store or serve.

CRISPY COOKIES

AMARETTI COOKIES

Servings Provided: 16

Prep & Cook Time: 30 minutes

Macro Counts - Per Serving:

- Calories: 86

- Net Carbohydrates: 1 g

- Fat Content: 8 g

- Protein: 2.5 g

Essential Ingredients:

- Coconut flour (2 tbsp.)

- Almond flour (1 cup)

- Erythritol (.5 cup)

- Baking powder (.5 tsp.)

- Cinnamon (.25 tsp.)

- Salt (.5 tsp.)

- Eggs (2)

- Vanilla extract (.5 tsp.)

- Coconut oil (4 tbsp.)

- Almond extract (.5 tsp.)

- Sugar-free jam (2 tbsp.)

- Shredded coconut (1 tbsp.)

Preparation Technique:

1. Cover a baking tray using a sheet of parchment baking paper.

2. Warm the oven to reach 400° F/204° C. Combine all of the dry fixings. After combining, work in the wet ones.

3. Shape into 16 cookies. Make a dent in the center of each one and bake for 15-17 minutes.

4. Let them cool a few minutes before adding a dab of jam to each one and a sprinkle of the coconut bits to serve.

COCONUT ALMOND COOKIES

Servings Provided: 6

Prep & Cook Time: 25-30 minutes

Macro Counts - Per Serving:

- Calories: 271

- Net Carbohydrates: 2 g

- Fat Content: 25 g

- Protein: 7 g

Essential Ingredients:

- Almond flour (1.25 cups)

- Unsweetened shredded coconut (.5 cup)

- Large eggs (3)

- Softened butter (6 tbsp.)

- Sugar substitute (.33 cup)

- Almond extract (1 tsp.)

- Ground cinnamon (.25 tsp.)

- Sea salt (.25 tsp.)

Preparation Technique:

1. Heat the oven to reach 350° F/177° C.

2. Spritz a baking tin with some cooking oil spray.

3. Combine the sweetener of choice and softened butter.

4. One at a time, whisk and stir in the eggs until well incorporated.

5. Stir in the rest of the fixings – with the coconut added last.

6. Drop by the spoonful onto the prepared baking tray to bake for 12 to 15 minutes.

7. When done, arrange them on a cooling rack to reach room temp before storing them.

CREAM CHEESE COOKIES

Servings Provided: 75 cookies @ 4 per serving

Prep & Cook Time: 20-23 minutes

Macro Counts - Per Serving:

- Calories: 204

- Net Carbohydrates: 2 g

- Fat Content: 19 g

- Protein: 4 g

Essential Ingredients:

- Surkin:1 or your favorite sugar substitute (.75 cup)
- Softened cream cheese (4 oz.)
- Butter (1 cup)
- Egg (1)
- Coconut flour (.5 cup)
- Almond flour (2 cups)

Preparation Technique:

1. Set the oven temperature to reach 350° F/177° C.

2. Cream the sweetener and butter until fluffy.

3. Fold in the cream cheese and add the egg.

4. Stir in both flours and mix in the vanilla.

5. Chill the prepared dough for a minimum of four hours.

6. Squeeze the dough into a cookie press. You can also roll it into a log and slice.

7. Bake them for eight to ten minutes for pressed cookies or 10-12 minutes – sliced.

GINGER SNAP COOKIES

Servings Provided: 1

Prep & Cook Time: 18-20 minutes

Macro Counts - Per Serving:

- Calories: 74

- Net Carbohydrates: 2.2 g

- Fat Content: 7 g

- Protein: 2.3 g

Essential Ingredients:

- Ground cloves (.25 tsp.)

- Nutmeg - .25 tsp.)

- Salt (.25 tsp.)

- Almond flour (2 cups)

- Ground cinnamon (.5 tsp.)

- Unsalted butter (.25 cup)

- Vanilla extract (1 tsp.)

- Large egg (1)

Preparation Technique:

1. Heat the oven temperature until it reaches 350° F/177° C.

2. Sift or whisk the dry components in a mixing bowl. Blend in the rest of the ingredients into the dry mixture using a hand blender. The dough will be stiff.

3. Measure out the dough for each cookie and flatten with a fork or your fingers.

4. Bake for about 9-11 minutes or until browned.

CHAPTER 11

CELIAC RECIPES - GLUTEN-FREE

If you suffer from the Celiac immune disease and cannot eat gluten, you realize it will damage your small intestine. The gluten protein is found in rye, barley, and wheat. You have a collection of delicious recipes in this segment to enjoy, even though you may find others within your new cookbook. So, cook your way to a healthier routine of dining.

BLACKBERRY LEMON MUFFINS

Servings Provided: 12

Prep & Cook Time: 45 minutes

Macro Counts - Per Serving:

- Calories: 277

- Net Carbohydrates: 5 g

- Fat Content: 25 g

- Protein: 8 g

Essential Ingredients:

- Almond flour (2 cups)

- Sea salt (.125 tsp.)

- G-F aluminum-free baking powder (2 tsp.)

- Coconut flour (1 tbsp.)

- Heavy cream (.5 cup)

- Unchilled eggs (2 large)

- Melted butter (.25 cup)

- Lemon juice (1 tbsp.) & zest (1 lemon)

- Pure vanilla extract (1 tsp.)

- Liquid stevia (12 drops)

- Fresh firm blackberries or cherries - fresh or frozen (1.5 cups)

- Chopped pecans (.5 cup)

Preparation Technique:

1. Set the oven temperature to reach 350° F/177° C.

2. Prepare a muffin pan with paper liners.

3. Mix the baking powder, almond flour, and salt into a food processor.

4. Pour in the cream, eggs, lemon juice, butter, lemon zest, vanilla, and stevia. Blend until creamy. Fold in the blackberries and pecans.

5. Empty the mixture into the muffin tins and set a timer to bake for 30 to 35 minutes.

6. Notes: If you are using frozen berries, do not defrost before adding to the recipe.

7. If you do not have a food processor, use an electric mixer.

8. Cool in the tins before removing.

BUTTER BREAD

Servings Provided: 1 loaf/8 servings

Prep & Cook Time: 40 minutes

Macro Counts - Per Serving:

- Calories: 243

- Net Carbohydrates: 2 g

- Fat Content: 20 g

- Protein: 10 g

Essential Ingredients:

- Fine ground almond flour (1.5 cups)

- G-F baking powder (2 tsp.)

- Fine-grain salt (1 tsp.)

- Melted butter (.25 cup)

- Large eggs (6)

- Cream of tartar (⅛ tsp.)

Preparation Technique:

1. Grease a baking loaf pan.

2. Beat the eggs until frothy.

3. Mix in the rest of the fixings.

4. Scoop the mixture into the pan.

5. Bake at 375° F/191° C for about ½ hour.

CLOUD AKA OOPSIE BREAD

Servings Provided: 10

Prep & Cook Time: 40 minutes

Macro Counts - Per Serving:

- Calories: 35

- Net Carbohydrates: 0.4 g

- Fat Content: 2.8 g

- Protein: 2.2 g

Essential Ingredients:

- Unchilled eggs (3)

- Unchilled cream cheese (3 tbsp.)

- Cream of tartar (.25 tsp.)

- Salt (.25 tsp.)

- Optional: Unflavored Whey Protein Powder - ex. - Perfect Keto (1 scoop)

Preparation Technique:

1. Set the oven temperature to 300° F/149° C.

2. Line two baking trays using a layer of parchment baking paper.

3. Separate the egg whites from the yolks, placing them into individual dishes.

4. Combine the egg yolks with the cream cheese using a hand mixer until well-combined.

5. Use the mixer to blend the egg whites with the cream of tartar and salt. Use the high-speed setting until stiff peaks form.

6. Slowly pour the yolk mixture into the egg whites and carefully fold until there are no white streaks.

7. Scoop the batter mix onto the baking tray about 0.5-.75-inches tall and about five inches apart.

8. Place the pan on the center oven rack. Bake until they're as desired (½ hour).

9. Slightly cool before slicing, or they will crumble.

CRANBERRY BREAD

Servings Provided: 12

Prep & Cook Time: 1 hour 50 minutes

Macro Counts - Per Serving:

- Calories: 179

- Net Carbohydrates: 4.7 g

- Fat Content: 15 g

- Protein: 6.4 g

Essential Ingredients:

- Almond flour (2 cups)

- Powdered erythritol or Swerve (.5 cup)

- Bak. powder (1.5 tsp.)

- Steviva stevia powder (.5 tsp.)

- Salt (1 tsp.)

- Bak. soda (.5 tsp.)

- Unsalted butter melted or coconut oil (4 tbsp.)

- Eggs at room temperature (4 large)

- Coconut milk (.5 cup)

- Cranberries (12 oz. bag)

- *Optional*: Honey or maple syrup - sub for Blackstrap molasses (1 tsp.)

- Also Needed: 9x5-inch loaf pan

Preparation Technique:

1. Heat the oven temperature to reach 350° F/177° C.

2. Lightly oil/grease the baking pan.

3. Sift the flour with the baking soda, erythritol/stevia, baking powder, and salt.

4. In another container, whisk the eggs, butter, honey, and coconut milk.

5. Combine it all until well combined.

6. Fold in the rinsed cranberries and add to the pan.

7. Bake it for about 1.25 hours. Watch the bread closely when you approach the one-hour marker since oven temperatures vary.

8. Transfer the pan to a wire rack to cool (15 min.) before removing from the pan.

90-SECOND ALMOND FLOUR BREAD

Servings Provided: 2 slices

Prep & Cook Time: 3 minutes

Macro Counts - Per Serving:

- Calories: 150

- Net Carbohydrates: 1 g

- Fat Content: 13 g

- Protein: 5 g

Essential Ingredients:

- Butter (1 tbsp.) **

- Blanched almond flour (3 tbsp.)

- Gluten-free bak.powder (.5 tsp.)

- Sea salt (1 pinch)

- Psyllium husk powder (1 tsp.)

- Egg (1 large)

Preparation Technique:

1. Melt the butter/ghee/coconut oil in a small glass rectangular container.

2. Meanwhile, whisk the flour with the baking powder, psyllium husk powder, and sea salt.

3. Add the flour mixture to the melted butter, and whisk, stirring until smooth.

4. Bake for about 15 minutes at 350° F/177° C, until firm. Alternately, Microwave for about 90 seconds, until firm. Run a knife along the edges. Flip the bread onto a plate or paper towel to release.

5. Slice it in half to form two thick slices. You can slice each piece in half for a thinner slice if desired.

6. Toast in a toaster for best results to improve its texture and reduce any eggy flavor.

7. ** Use ghee or coconut oil for dairy-free in place of the butter.

KETO SANDWICH ROLLS - DAIRY & GLUTEN-FREE

Servings Provided: 4 buns

Prep & Cook Time: 45 minutes

Macro Counts - Per Serving:

- Calories: 306

- Net Carbohydrates: 3 g

- Fat Content: 26 g

- Protein: 9 g

Essential Ingredients:

- Almond flour (1 cup)

- Bak. powder (1 tsp.)

- Psyllium husk powder (2 tbsp.)

- Raw sunflower seeds/or another unsalted seed (2 tsp.)

- White sesame seeds (1 tsp.)

- Chia seeds (1 tsp.)

- Black sesame seeds (1 tsp.)

- Erythritol (1 tsp.)

- Sea salt (.25 tsp.)

- Apple cider/white vinegar (1 tbsp.)

- Eggs (2 large)

- Salted butter/coconut oil (3 tbsp.)

- Rapidly boiling water (.25 cup)

Preparation Technique:

1. Warm the oven in advance to reach 350° F/177° C.

2. Sift or whisk each of the dry ingredients until combined, removing all lumps.

3. In another container, mix all of the wet fixings (omit the boiling water until step 5).

4. Pour the wet into the dry mixture to give the appearance of thick nut butter.

5. Pour in the *boiling* water and mix. The dough will be sticky.

6. Portion the sticky dough into four sections/rolls, and place on a parchment covered baking tray. Use a mixing spoon to place them on the baking sheet. Form them into a bun shape with oiled hands as necessary.

7. Bake for 35 minutes. They should have a hollow sound when tapped on the bottom.

8. Cool and slice for sandwiches or burgers. Store in an airtight container or bag.

SAVORY GLUTEN-FREE BREAD ROLLS

Servings Provided: 8

Prep & Cook Time: 36 minutes

Macro Counts - Per Serving:

- Calories: 216

- Net Carbohydrates: 4 g

- Fat Content: 16 g

- Protein: 11 g

Essential Ingredients:

- Shredded mozzarella cheese - Part-skim low moisture (1.5 cups)

- Cream cheese - Full-fat (2 ounces)

- Almond flour (1.33 cups)

- Coconut flour (2 tablespoons)

- Double-acting & aluminum-free baking powder (1.5 tablespoons)

- Large eggs (3) 1 egg is reserved for egg wash

Preparation Technique:

1. Set the oven temperature setting to 350° F/177° C. Prepare a baking tray using a sheet of baking paper.

2. Whisk the coconut flour with the almond flour and baking powder.

3. Toss the cream cheese and mozzarella into a microwave-safe dish. Cover and melt in the microwave using 30-second intervals.

4. Stir the cheese until it's completely melted (1 min.). Cool slightly and combine with two eggs, and the almond flour mixture in a food processor with a dough blade attachment.

5. Pulse using the high speed until it's blended (sticky is okay).

6. Scoop the dough onto a large sheet of plastic wrap. Knead a few times until you create a smooth ball.

7. Divide the dough into eight parts. Shape and place the balls onto the baking sheet about two inches apart.

8. Whisk the final egg and brush the rolls with the egg wash.

9. Bake the rolls using the middle oven rack for 20-25 minutes. They're best eaten while hot.

3 INGREDIENT LOW-CARB - GLUTEN-FREE CREPES

Servings Provided: 6

Prep & Cook Time: 8-10 minutes

Macro Counts - Per Serving:

- Calories: 103

- Net Carbohydrates: 1.2 g

- Fat Content: 6.6 g

- Protein: 7.3 g

Essential Ingredients:

- Cream cheese full fat (4 tbsp.)

- Eggs (4 whole + 4 whites)

- Psyllium husk (2 tbsp.) or Psyllium husk powder (1 tbsp.)

- For Frying: Butter (as needed)

Preparation Technique:

1. Toss all fixings into a food processor/power blender or with a stick blender. The batter will be very thin.

2. Warm butter in a large skillet. Pour in some batter and swirl it around until it is evenly distributed.

3. Fry using the medium temperature setting until the top has firmed. Flip it over and fry until it is browned as desired. Continue until all batter is used.

YEAST BREAD

Servings Provided: 12 slices

Prep & Cook Time: 1 hour 5 minutes

Macro Counts - Per Serving:

- Calories: 226

- Net Carbohydrates: 0 g

- Fat Content: 19 g

- Protein: 8 g

Essential Ingredients:

- Active dry yeast (2 tsp.)

- Inulin (2 tsp.)

- Warm water - must be ** 105° F/41° C – 110° F/43° C - *SUPER IMPORTANT* (1 cup)

- Almond flour (2 cups)

- Coconut flour (2 tbsp.)

- Fine - flaxseed meal (.75 cup)

- Sour cream/cottage cheese (.25 cup)

- Psyllium husk - finely ground (2 tbsp.)

- Xanthan gum (2 tsp.)

- Bak. powder (2 tsp.)

- Salt (1 tsp.)

- Cream of tartar (.25 tsp.)

- Eggs (2)

- Melted & cooled butter (.25 cup)

- Apple cider vinegar (1 tbsp.)

- Optional: Erythritol (1 tbsp.)

- Also Needed 8x4-inch bread pan

Preparation Technique:

1. Lightly oil the baking pan.

2. Combine the yeast with the inulin and warm water (**105° F/41° C to – 110° F/43° C) in a cereal-sized bowl, mixing using a fork until the yeast is somewhat dissolved. This is important! The inulin feeds the yeast just like sugar does in traditional recipes. (Use sugar if you don't have this.) It won't cause the carbs to increase because the yeast eats the sugar and converts it to carbon dioxide.

3. Allow the bowl of yeast water to rest/stand for ten minutes while measuring the other ingredients. As it works, it will bubble and increase in size, which is called proofing.

4. Combine all of the dry fixings in a large mixing container and set it to the side.

5. Add all of the wet ingredients (minus the yeast mixture)into another container and mix until thoroughly combined.

6. Once the yeast is proofed, mix it into the bowl of dry components and then into the bowl of wet ingredients. (Unfortunately, if it doesn't bubble or grow, your yeast is dead, and you'll need fresh yeast.)

7. Scoop the bread dough into the loaf pan and smooth the top.

8. Proof the dough in a warm space until the dough has risen just past the pan's top (50-60 min.).

9. Meanwhile, warm the oven to 350° F/177 ° C.

10. Gently transfer the loaf pan to the oven. Bake for 50 minutes to one hour or until golden brown. Keep an eye on the bread and cover with a foil dome if it starts to get too brown after 40 minutes.

11. Cool the bread in the pan until you can safely remove it without burning your hands (20 min.). It will deflate a lot if you handle it while still hot.

12. Do not slice until entirely cool for best results.

13. Store at room temp in an airtight bag or covered with foil for up to five days. It's incredible for sandwiches.

CHAPTER 12

EXTRA-SPECIAL CAKES & CUPCAKES

CAKES

CARROT CAKE

Servings Provided: 16

Prep & Cook Time: 1.5 hours

Macro Counts - Per Serving:

- Calories: 370

- Net Carbohydrates: 2 g

- Fat Content: 35 g

- Protein: 8 g

Essential Ingredients:

- Almond flour (2.75 cups)

- Unsweetened shredded coconut (1 cup)

- Powdered Swerve (1.25 cups)

- Gluten-free baking powder (2 tsp.)

- Cinnamon (2 tsp.)

- Salt (.5 tsp.)

- Eggs (6 large)

- Avocado oil (.5 cup)

- Coconut milk (.25 cup)

- Grated carrots (2 cups)

- Vanilla extract (1 tbsp.)

- Pecan pieces (.5 cup) *The Icing*:

- Cream cheese (8 oz. block)

- Powdered Swerve (1 cup)

- Heavy whipping cream (.5 cup)

- Coconut extract (1 tsp.)

- Pecan pieces (.5 cup)

Preparation Technique:

1. Warm the oven temperature to 350° F/177° C.

2. Grease a 10.5-inch cast-iron skillet well or line the bottom with a piece of parchment paper.

3. Combine all of the cake ingredients in a large mixing container until smooth. Pour the batter into the prepared skillet.

4. Transfer to the oven and bake for one hour, covering with foil at the 45-minute mark. Cool it thoroughly.

5. For the frosting, combine the cream cheese, swerve, and heavy whipping cream in a medium mixing container. Beat with a hand mixer on high until light and fluffy. Ice the cake then sprinkle with pecan pieces.

6. Refrigerate until ready to serve.

CHOCOLATE ROLL CAKE

Servings Provided: 12

Prep & Cook Time: 25 minutes

Macro Counts - Per Serving:

- Calories: 275

- Net Carbohydrates: 3 g

- Fat Content: 25 g

- Protein: 5 g

Essential Ingredients:

The Mix:

- Almond flour (1 cup)

- Psyllium husk powder (.25 cup)

- Baking powder (1 tsp.)

- Cocoa powder (.25 cup)

- Erythritol (.25 cup)

- Melted butter (4 tbsp.)

- Eggs (3)

- Coconut milk (.25 cup)

- Sour cream (.25 cup)

- Vanilla (1 tsp.)

The Filling:

- Cream cheese (8 oz. pkg.)

- Butter (8 tbsp.)

- Sour cream (.25 cup)

- Erythritol (.25 cup)

- Stevia (.25 tsp.)

- Vanilla (1 tsp.)

Preparation Technique:

1. Heat the oven in advance (350° F/177° C). 181

2. Combine each of the dry fixings and mix slowly with the wet components.

3. Spread the dough over a foil-covered baking tin to bake (12-15 min.). Transfer to the counter to cool slightly to handle.

4. Prepare the filling. Spread the mixture over the dough and roll up your cake. Be sure to make it tight and serve when desired.

CUPCAKES & MUG CAKES

BLUEBERRY CUPCAKES

Servings Provided: 12

Prep & Cook Time: 26-30 minutes

Macro Counts - Per Serving:

- Calories: 138

- Net Carbohydrates: 2.8 g

- Fat Content: 11 g

- Protein: 4.4 g

Essential Ingredients:

- Melted butter (1 stick)

- Granulated sweetener of choice (4 tbsp./as desired)

- Coconut flour (.5 cup)

- Baking powder (1 tsp.)

- Lemon juice (2 tbsp.)

- Vanilla (1 tsp.)

- Lemon zest (2 tbsp.)

- Eggs (8 medium)

- Fresh blueberries (1 cup)

Preparation Technique:

1. Set the oven temp to preheat at 350° F/177° C.

2. Melt and mix the butter with the sweetener, coconut flour, baking powder, vanilla, lemon juice, and zest together in a large mixing container.

3. Break and add in the eggs. Mix thoroughly as you prepare the batter.

4. Taste the cupcake batter to ensure you have used enough sweetener and flavors.

5. Portion the batter into the tins. Press in a few fresh blueberries in the batter of each cupcake.

6. Bake for 15 minutes, or until golden on the outside, and cooked in the center.

7. Cover with sugar-free cream cheese frosting; vanilla or lemon flavor is perfect. Garnish with fresh blueberries and lemon zest. (Icing/frosting is additional and optional.)

CHOCOLATE MUG CAKE

Servings Provided: 1 large

Prep & Cook Time: 6 minutes

Macro Counts - Per Serving:

- Calories: 473

- Net Carbohydrates: 5.2 g

- Fat Content: 38 g

- Protein: 13.7 g

Essential Ingredients:

- Butter (1 tbsp.)

- Unsweetened Baking Chocolate Bar - ex. Baker's (1 oz.)

- Swerve - The Ultimate Icing Sugar Replacement (4 tbsp.)

- Baking powder (.5 tsp.)

- Salt (1 pinch)

- Almond flour (2 tbsp.)

- 100% Cocoa Special Dark - ex. Hershey's (1 tsp.)

- Egg (1 large)

- Vanilla extract (.25 tsp.)

Preparation Technique:

1. Melt the butter and chocolate by microwaving at ½ minute intervals or until completely melted in a tall coffee mug.

2. Mix in the baking powder, almond flour, sweetener, salt, and cocoa powder.

3. Add the egg and vanilla extract. Mix with a spoon until completely blended.

4. Microwave for 50 seconds to one minute.

5. Serve with whipped cream and a dusting of cocoa powder.

SPICE CAKES

Servings Provided: 12

Prep & Cook Time: Under ½ hour

Macro Counts - Per Serving:

- Calories: 277

- Net Carbohydrates: 3 g

- Fat Content: 27 g

- Protein: 6 g

Essential Ingredients:

- Salted butter (.5 cup)

- Erythritol (.75 cup)

- Eggs (4 - divided)

- Vanilla extract (1 tsp.)

- Ground clove (.25 tsp.)

- Allspice (.5 tsp.)

- Nutmeg (.5 tsp.)

- Almond flour (2 cups)

- Baking powder (2 tsp.)

- Cinnamon (.5 tsp.)

- Ginger (.5 tsp.)

- Water (5 tbsp.)

- Also Needed: Cupcake tray

Preparation Technique:

1. Set the oven temperature to 350° F/177° C.

2. Prepare the baking tray with liners (12).

3. Mix the butter and erythritol with a hand mixer. Once it's smooth, combine with two eggs and the vanilla. Add the rest of the eggs and mix well.

4. Grind the clove to a fine powder and add with the rest of the spices. Whisk into the mixture. Stir in the baking powder and almond flour. Blend in the water. When the

5. Bake for 15 minutes. Cool slightly to serve.

CONCLUSION

I hope you have thoroughly enjoyed every chapter of *Keto Bread Cookbook.* I also hope it provided you with all of the tools you need to achieve your goals as you pass through the ketogenic plan phases baking fresh homemade bread.

You have the basics of what the plan is, but now it's time to understand some of the method's pitfalls. However, each of the issues is an indication that your body is in ketosis. These are a few of the signs you will observe as you begin the transition.

You may experience the 'keto flu' or 'induction flu,' which involves lowered mental functions and energy. You may suffer from sleeping issues, bouts of nausea, increased hunger, or other possible digestive worries. Several days into the plan should remedy these effects. If not, add ½ teaspoon of salt to a glass of water and drink it to help with the side effects. You may need to do this once a day in the first week, and it could take about 15 to 20 minutes before it helps. It will go away!

Leg cramps may be an issue as you begin ketosis. The loss of magnesium (a mineral) can be a demon and create a bit of pain with the onset of the keto diet plan changes. With the loss of the minerals during urination, you could experience bouts of cramps in your legs.

You may also notice an aroma similar to nail polish. Not surprising because this is acetone, a ketone product. It may also give you a unique body odor as your body adjusts to the diet changes. Maintain good oral health and use a breath refresher if needed. The side effects don't have the same impact on every person. These are merely guidelines for you to better understand how the dieting techniques may work for you.

Finally, if you found this book useful in any way, a review on Amazon is always appreciated!

9 798578 500558